COMBATING MEMORY LOSS

Common Problems & Treatments

2011 Report

A Special Report published by the editors of
Mind, Mood & Memory
in conjunction with
Massachusetts General Hospital
Boston, Massachusetts

Combating Memory Loss: Common Problems & Treatments

Consulting Editors: M. Cornelia Cremens, MD, MPH, Director of Inpatient Geriatric Psychiatry Consultation, Division of Psychiatry and Medicine, Massachusetts General Hospital; Assistant Professor of Psychiatry, Harvard Medical School William Falk, MD, Director of Outpatient Geriatric Psychiatry, Massachusetts General Hospital, Assistant Professor of Psychiatry, Harvard Medical School

Author: Stephanie Watson
Group Directors, Belvoir Media Group: Diane Muhlfeld, Jay Roland
Creative Director, Belvoir Media Group: Judi Crouse
Contributing Editor: Susan Jimison Vitek

Publisher, Belvoir Media Group: Timothy H. Cole

ISBN: 1-879620-88-X

To order additional copies of this report or for customer service questions, please call 877-300-0253 or write to Health Special Reports, 800 Connecticut Avenue, Norwalk, CT 06854-1631.

This publication is intended to provide readers with accurate and timely medical news and information. It is not intended to give personal medical advice, which should be obtained directly from a physician. We regret that we cannot respond to individual inquiries about personal health matters.

Report on Combating Memory Loss
Common Problems & Treatments

Memory problems are common as we age. Often simple forgetfulness is brought on by normal wear and tear on the brain. But for some people, a fading memory may be an indication of physical problems—such as thyroid problems or nutritional deficiencies—or neurological disorders affecting cognition—such as Alzheimer's disease, Parkinson's disease, or vascular dementia. These are not normal accompaniments to aging, and they require treatment.

This report will help you understand how normal memory works, and why it is important to everyday functioning. It will cover factors that interfere with memory and suggest steps that may help you overcome them and strengthen your powers of recall. It also will describe memory problems that require medical intervention, and provide information on risk factors, symptoms and available treatments.

In this report, you'll find ways to help protect yourself against memory loss from Alzheimer's disease and other forms of dementia, and improve your ability to cope with memory lapses. Finally, the report will highlight the latest research findings that may one day lead to advances in the diagnosis and treatment of memory disorders.

■ ■ ■

HIGHLIGHTS

■ Scientists use brain scans to "read" memory (Page 14, Box 1-2).

■ Study: Sharpest seniors have fewer brain tangles likened to AD (Page 18, Box 2-2).

■ Vigorous exercise may improve MCI (Page 19, Box 2-3).

■ Diabetes speeds progression of MCI (Page 19, Box 2-4).

■ Apathy, agitation, depression linked to faster cognitive decline (Page 23, Box 2-5).

■ Analysis calls research on smoking and AD into question (Page 22, Box 3-2).

■ High levels of an inflammation indicator linked with thinking problems (Page 23, Box 3-3).

■ Diabetes trebles risk of dementia among people with MCI (Page 28, Box 3-4).

■ Severe sleep apnea may cause brain damage (Page 30, Box 3-5).

■ Vitamin D deficiency linked to cognitive impairment in women (Page 32, Box 3-6).

■ Mild Parkinsonian signs linked to increased dementia risk (Page 33, Box 3-7).

■ Treatment that cures heart arrhythmia appears to lower Alzheimer's risk (Page 34, Box 3-9).

■ Most people unaware they've suffered a "silent stroke" (Page 35, Box 3-10).

■ Exposure to pesticides can boost risk of Alzheimer's (Page 36, Box 3-11).

HIGHLIGHTS
continued from previous page

- MGH study: Protein associated with AD may be part of the immune system (Page 37, Box 3-12).

- Thinking and memory problems may indicate higher stroke risk (Page 43, Box 4-5).

- Chromium picolinate supplements may improve cognition (Page 46, Box 4-6).

- Memory decline gets worse with stress (Page 48, Box 4-7).

- Scans find differences in glucose metabolism in early- vs. late-onset AD (Page 52, Box 5-2).

- Animal study provides new evidence for an Alzheimer's smell test (Page 54, Box 5-3).

- Finding may lead to eye test for Alzheimer's disease (Page 55, Box 5-4)

- Fish oil supplements may improve memory (Page 63, Box 6-1).

- AD drug Dimebon fails in Phase III trial (Page 65, Box 7-1).

- Immunoglobulin treatment slows progression of Alzheimer's (Page 67, Box 7-2).

- New biomarker measures effectiveness of AD drug bapineuzumab (Page 69, 7-3).

- New theory of Alzheimer's may call drug research into question (Page 70, Box 7-4).

- First gene study for Alzheimer's disease gets underway (Page 71, Box 7-5).

- Dietary magnesium boosts short- and long-term memory (Page 77, Box 8-2).

- Gene increases risk for both obesity and dementia (Page 79, Box 8-4).

- Physical strength linked to lower Alzheimer's risk (Page 80, Box 8-5).

- Exercise lowers risk of mild cognitive impairment (Page 81, Box 8-6).

- Sleep loss affects remembering and quality of decisions (Page 84, Box 8-10).

- Meaningful social involvement may improve cognitive functioning (Page 86, Box 8-12).

- Scientists find visual evidence of effects of learning on brain (Page 89, Box 8-14).

- Regular meditation may reverse memory loss (Page 92, Box 9-2).

TABLE OF CONTENTS

Combating Memory Loss
2011 Report

ABOUT MASSACHUSETTS GENERAL HOSPITAL

Founded in 1811, Massachusetts General Hospital (MGH) is the third-oldest general hospital in the United States and the oldest and largest teaching hospital of Harvard Medical School. MGH offers world-renowned diagnostic and therapeutic care in virtually every specialty of medicine and surgery. Pursuing its three-part mission of patient care, teaching, and research, the hospital is consistently ranked among the top hospitals nationwide. It houses the most prolific hospital-based research program in the country, with an annual budget of almost $550 million. The hospital's Department of Psychiatry has been ranked No. 1 for 13 straight years by *U.S. News & World Report*. The department's Geriatric Neurobehavioral Clinic and Gerontology Research Unit provide comprehensive clinical care and research for Alzheimer's disease and other neurodegenerative disorders. ■

INTRODUCTION

As we grow older, our fear of losing our memories grows, too. Many of us worry that our momentary lapses and frustrating mental blanks are the first indications of dreaded dementia—severe memory loss that affects personality and behavior, and interferes with normal activities of daily functioning. A large national survey of 1,008 adults conducted by the Metlife Foundation found that for people over 55, Alzheimer's outranked cancer, heart disease, diabetes and stroke as the most feared disease. What will happen, we worry, if we keep our physical health in old age, but lose our minds?

Although these fears may be understandable, they also may be unnecessary for the majority of us. While it's true that the likelihood of developing dementia increases with age, only about 30 to 40 percent of people in their 70s and 80s have dementia. With a brain-benefiting lifestyle including exercise and a healthy diet, chances are good you can remain mentally alert well into advanced old age.

There are a number of causes of memory loss that have nothing to do with dementia, and these often can be addressed with proper diagnosis and treatment. But even for those who have progressive neurological disorders, the outlook is improving. As researchers come closer to understanding the causes of Alzheimer's disease (AD) and other dementias, new treatment approaches become possible. Scientists are developing new diagnostic techniques and devising medications and therapies that may one day prevent or perhaps even reverse serious memory loss.

Still, memory loss is a cause for concern. According to the Alzheimer's Association, about one out of eight people age 65 and older has AD, which affects an estimated 5.3 million Americans. The number of new cases per year is expected to grow to 615,000 by 2030. Currently, someone in America develops AD every 70 seconds, and direct and indirect costs amount to more than $172 billion each year, according to the *2010 Alzheimer's Disease Facts and Figures* report published by the Alzheimer's Association. Other disorders such as vascular dementia—the second most common form of primary dementia, often caused by stroke—add to the burden.

The broader social impact of this tidal wave of memory troubles is enormous, and so is the personal toll on patients and families. Failing memory can lead to increased dependence and loss of self-esteem. Beyond that, it can strike at the root of who we are as individuals. If we cannot manage basic activities on our own or recognize our friends and family, if we have no memory of our life's experiences, how can we be truly ourselves?

It's understandable, then, that when our memory slips, we have questions: Is this normal age-related memory loss, or a sign of something more serious? Can anything be done to prevent, stop or reverse fading memory abilities? What other factors might cause memory decline? What options are available if memory loss turns out to be progressive?

The following pages should help answer these questions and many more. They will cover memory loss from every angle, providing the knowledge you need to understand how memory works and why forgetfulness develops. They will describe current techniques for diagnosis and treatment of dementia, recommend strategies you can use to avoid memory loss, and share the latest research. Finally, they'll cover new drugs in the pipeline that may one day help to prevent, slow or even reverse the progress of neurocognitive disease—making it possible for you to forget your worries about memory loss. ■

1 WHAT IS MEMORY?

All animals and humans have memory. Essentially, memory is the way we store information until we need it.

Some people are naturally better than others at remembering, but how they got that way stems from two separate factors. Genetics accounts for about half of our memory—some people may be born with the ability to retain easily what they learn, while others may have to work harder. The other half of memory is shaped by our environment. Factors such as diet, education, and medical care all combine to affect brain function. Whether it is possible, even if you weren't blessed with a strong memory, to "train your brain" by stimulating it with flash cards, reasoning and problem-solving games, and other intellectual activities is still open to debate. But there is evidence that mental activity, social involvement and physical exercise may be associated with better memory performance.

How memory works

Imagine that you're taking a stroll in New York City and spot a street performer juggling a dozen fire-tipped pins. The performer is so amazing that you want to call your grandkids and tell them about him—but you've forgotten your cell phone.

In order to describe what you saw to your grandchildren, you'll need to create a memory. Your sensory organs have gathered information about the street performer—from his bright-orange wig to the smell of the fire emanating from his juggling pins. Now the memory process begins.

Memory has three distinct phases: encoding, storage, and retrieval. As you were watching the street performer, your eyes, ears and nose were transmitting information via neurons to the regions of your brain that are associated with sight, sound, and smell. The impulses sped from one nerve cell to another across tiny gaps called synapses. Each of the individual cues was combined into a single memory in a region of your brain called the hippocampus (see Box 1-1). This process is known as encoding.

Next came the storage phase of the process. Your hippocampus sent the memory to the cerebral cortex, a kind of permanent file cabinet where it can remain for a long period of time.

There are two distinct mechanisms to memory storage: *short-term* (working) *memory*, and *long-term memory*. Short-term memory is the information that your mind stores for immediate recall. Your short-term memory can hold small amounts of information for limited amounts of time. So if you had walked a few steps down the road to a pay phone and called your grandchildren to tell them about the street performer, you would have been using your short-term memory.

Long-term memory involves retaining information for days, months, or years. When you recall the street performer at your niece's birthday party six months after the event, you are using your long-term memory. The brain can store almost limitless amounts of long-term memory, which is why we can learn so many new things and retain what we've learned for many years.

BOX 1-1: THE BRAIN'S MEMORY CENTERS

PREFRONTAL CORTEX
Located in the cortical regions of the frontal lobe, this area is believed to store short-term memories and is thought to be involved in planning complex cognitive functions.

CEREBRAL CORTEX
Stores memories for long periods of time. Functions like a permanent file cabinet.

HIPPOCAMPUS
This region of the brain encodes visual, sound, taste, touch, and smell cues from other parts of the brain into memories.

PARAHIPPOCAMPAL CORTEX
Part of the temporal lobe on the pathway to the hippocampus, it is active in memory retrieval.

Long-term memories come in different forms. The color of your mother's hair, the sum of two plus two, and the name of the first U.S. president are semantic memories. They are general facts. Episodic memories capture the sights, sounds, and emotions of specific places and events: the joy you felt when you scored the winning run in the championship Little League game, the smell of your aunt's 80th birthday cake candles, or the pain you experienced when you fell off your bike and skinned your knee. Procedural memories are the skills you've picked up throughout your life, such as riding a bicycle, driving a car, and even getting dressed.

Recalling a memory

Suppose that your grandchildren came over to your house for dinner, and you were ready to recount that story of the talented street performer. Now the retrieval process would begin. When you retrieve information, you are literally pulling it from nerve pathways. You remember information as your brain reactivates the same pathway that was originally triggered when you stored the memory. This process can be fast or slow, depending on how familiar you are with the information and how well you learned it in the first place.

Memories can be retrieved via one of two processes: recall or recognition. In this case, you'll probably use recall to remember the street performer. Recall involves directly accessing the memory. You also use recall when you remember the name of the television show you watched last night. Recognition, on the other hand, uses cues to help you retrieve a memory. When you were in school, you used recognition every time you took a multiple-choice test.

Studying how normal memory works

Through the use of new technologies such as specialized scanning equipment, scientists are better able to study how the brain works. Many scientists believe that a memory is formed when a brief pattern of electrical impulses moves through a network of neurons, strengthening connections between the affected brain cells. This leaves a "memory trace" in the brain, which is revived when the information is recalled. The brain has many different areas, each of which specializes in different types of information. Researchers now know that certain attributes of a memory are grouped with other, similar recollections; for example, the smell of chocolate ice cream may be grouped with recollections of salt water taffy and popcorn. When you recall information, your brain cross-references the many different attributes of that memory.

Researchers have actually captured brain activity that indicates where certain memories are created and what the likelihood is that someone will be able to recall that information.

Scanning studies

Scientists at Massachusetts General Hospital's Nuclear Magnetic Resonance Center, Harvard, Washington University in St. Louis, and Stanford University used brain-scanning devices to record the instantaneous birth—and demise— of a memory. Participants in some studies were told to look at a list of words and classify them as either concrete (e.g.,"table") or abstract (e.g., "love") while their brain activity was observed with scanning. They were later asked to recall whether specific words had or had not been included in the list. Their answers indicated which words they had remembered and which they had forgotten. Researchers then compared levels of activity recorded in various parts of subjects' brains while they were classifying words they later remembered and words they later forgot.

The researchers found that words associated with high levels of activity in the left frontal lobe, located just behind the temple, and the left temporal lobe, situated behind the ear, were most likely to be remembered. Especially important was a part of the left temporal lobe called the parahippocampal cortex, which is on the pathway to the hippocampus, the part of the brain that is vital for storing and retrieving memories. Words associated with lower levels of activity were most likely to be forgotten.

In similar experiments testing visual memory conducted at Stanford University in California, researchers found that activity in the right prefrontal lobe and both the left and right temporal lobes predicts which pictures of scenes will be remembered. Once again, the largest region of activation occurred in the parahippocampal cortex.

Although it is not clear why participants remembered some words and scenes and forgot others, researchers suggested that the participants might have remembered a word or picture better when they connected it to their own experience. For example, a person who had traveled extensively to Western national parks might have recognized a scene from Bryce Canyon National Park, while another person might have dismissed the picture as just another desert scene.

Another scanning study has shed light on brain activity related to short-term memory. Researchers used functional magnetic resonance imaging (fMRI) scans to measure blood flow in the brains of volunteers as they tried to hold information in their minds for a brief period. (Increases in blood flow to a brain region indicate greater brain activity in that area.) Volunteers were asked to look at

Box 1-2: Scientists use brain scans to "read" memory

In a fascinating study that involved a sophisticated form of "mind reading," researchers succeeded in using functional magnetic resonance imaging (fMRI) to decode individual memories in the brains of volunteers and identify which of several distinct scenes they were recalling. The scientists showed three short film clips to a group of 10 participants. Each clip showed a different woman performing a series of simple, everyday actions. After they had viewed the films several times, study participants were placed in an fMRI machine and asked to recall each clip as vividly as possible as recordings of their brain activity were made. The participants were then asked to recall the film clips at random, and indicate on a key pad which film they had remembered. Researchers found that they were able to identify which of the three films was being recalled by distinct brain patterns associated with each of the three memory traces, according to a report on the study published in the March 11, 2010 online edition of *Current Biology*. What's more, the authors reported that the brain activity associated with remembering each clip was remarkably similar among all 10 participants.

images on a computer screen for one second and remember either the orientation of the image, or its color. After a 10-second delay following exposure to each image, they were shown a second image and asked to indicate if it was identical to the one they had been told to remember. Scans measured blood flow in the primary visual cortex—the area of the brain associated with processing visual stimuli—during exposure to the image, during the 10-second delay, and during the recall process.

Results revealed that volunteers recruited the same neural machinery while remembering as they did when they saw an original stimulus and that during the 10-second period when volunteers were holding information in short-term memory, the area of the visual cortex that was activated depended on what a study participant had been asked to remember. Brain areas responsible for remembering color were active when volunteers were asked to remember an object's color, but areas responsible for orientation were not; areas responsible for remembering orientation were active when volunteers were asked to remember orientation, while color areas were not. During the 10-second period in which information was held in short-term memory, the brain activation was so specific that researchers were able to decipher what volunteers were remembering by looking at where the activity took place. The findings suggest that while short-term memory is engaged, the brain is actively "thinking" about the information that must be remembered so that the information will be retained, but forgetting other details. The results, which were published in the February 2009 issue of *Psychological Science*, also suggest that people have voluntary control over what information they store in short-term memory.

In a more recent study, researchers succeeded in tracking complex episodic memories (recollections of everyday events) using fMRI scans, and were able to distinguish which of three possible scenes study participants were remembering by identifying patterns of activity in their hippocampi (see Box 1-2). ■

2 WHY AGING MINDS FORGET

All of us forget things from time to time. Occasional memory lapses are normal, and the memory problems experienced by most people who live well into old age are normal age-associated memory impairment (see Box 2-1).

Forgetting may even be part of a healthy memory system. Neuroscientists at Stanford University found that people actually block out certain memories so that they can remember more important things, much in the way that you might tune out the annoying drone sitting next to you at a dinner party so that you can focus on another, more interesting conversation.

The researchers tested 20 young men and women by having them study 40 word pairs comprised of a cue word (such as ATTIC) combined with one of six possible associate words (such as ATTIC/dust or ATTIC/junk). After sub-

BOX 2-1: MEMORY IMPAIRMENT STATISTICS

This chart shows the percent of U.S. men with moderate to severe memory impairment vs. the percent of U.S. women with moderate to severe memory impairment at age 65+, and also shows the progression of memory impairment by age ranges.

Overall, fewer than one in five adults over age 65 experiences moderate to severe memory impairment.

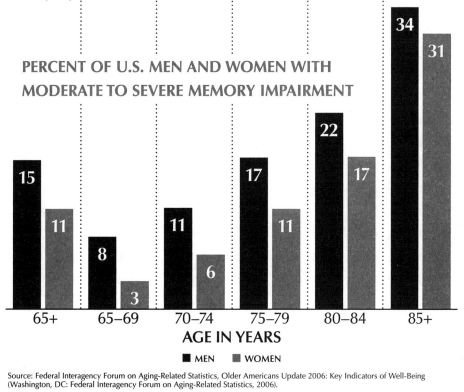

PERCENT OF U.S. MEN AND WOMEN WITH MODERATE TO SEVERE MEMORY IMPAIRMENT

AGE IN YEARS	MEN	WOMEN
65+	15	11
65–69	8	3
70–74	11	6
75–79	17	11
80–84	22	17
85+	34	31

■ MEN ■ WOMEN

Source: Federal Interagency Forum on Aging-Related Statistics, Older Americans Update 2006: Key Indicators of Well-Being (Washington, DC: Federal Interagency Forum on Aging-Related Statistics, 2006).

jects studied the word pairs, researchers asked them to remember one pair for each cue word, while consciously forgetting the other possible combinations. Functional magnetic resonance imaging (fMRI) of the subjects' brains showed that the prefrontal cortex was actively involved in the process of remembering one pair from among the competing pairs, and that this region became gradually less active as subjects concentrated on remembering the correct pair for a second or third time. Later tests showed that people who experienced the greatest decrease in prefrontal cortex activity were those who were most successful at "tuning out" the irrelevant words and recalling the correct word pair.

Although forgetting in some circumstances can be useful, at other times it can be frustrating, embarrassing, and inconvenient. If you've ever lost your car in the mall parking lot or spent an hour searching for your cell phone, you can relate.

Even when a memory is not totally forgotten, it can become less accurate. Just like any computer, the human brain isn't perfect. Sometimes memories can become distorted or misinterpreted. Important elements of a memory may disappear completely.

The good news is that most memory problems are not related to dementia. In the majority of individuals, the problem stems from physical or emotional issues, or from the normal effects of aging.

Dehydration, fever, head injury, low thyroid function, liver and kidney problems, high blood pressure, obesity, poor nutrition, low blood sugar, and reactions to medications all are physical factors that can cause temporary memory impairment (see Chapter 3 for more on the causes of memory loss). Fortunately, these conditions can be treated.

Emotional distress also can have a devastating effect on memory. Repeated stress, sleeplessness, depression, and anxiety can interfere with the normal encoding and storage process, and can significantly affect your ability to remember even the simplest things.

Age-associated memory impairment (AAMI)

In addition to the everyday memory loss caused by physical and emotional factors, the aging process can take a toll on memory. Age-associated memory impairment (AAMI) starts early in life and progresses with age. We begin to lose brain cells (neurons) in our late 20s, a few at a time, although people who remain healthy and are mentally, socially, and physically active are able to generate new cells to replace many of these lost neurons. Our bodies also produce lower levels of the chemicals brain cells need to work. The combination of fewer brain cells and lower levels of brain chemicals changes the way the brain stores information and makes it harder to recall stored information.

The brain actually shrinks as we get older, losing both volume and weight. The shrinkage is the result of the gradual loss of neurons, and damage to the branch-like dendrites and nerve fibers called axons that extend from the neurons, connecting them to other cells. One important study suggests that changes in the brain's "white matter"—the bundles of long, slender nerve fibers that project from neurons and enable them to communicate with other neurons— may be more to blame for age-associated memory decline than changes in the "gray matter"—areas in the brain's cortex composed of cell bodies of neurons that are responsible for most important memory functions.

The researchers scanned the brains of a group of 36 young adults (ages 18–28) and a group of 38 healthy older adults (ages 61–86) and used an advanced technique to measure the integrity of the bundles of nerve fibers, or white matter, that connected different regions within their brains. The scientists also administered a series of tests designed to measure memory and other mental processes. The researchers found that compared to younger subjects, the older subjects showed significantly more signs of thinning of the cortex and reduced white matter integrity. Tests showed that thinning of the gray matter was concentrated in areas associated with motor and sensory functions, while decreases in white matter density were widespread and affected many brain areas, including those associated with memory and cognition.

Participants' performance on tests was not correlated with gray matter thickness. It was, however, strongly correlated with white matter density, with lower density linked to lower test performance. The authors theorize that age-related changes in white matter density may result from degradation of the myelin sheath, a fatty covering that surrounds nerve fibers and ensures the efficient conduction of signals from cell to cell. The breakdown of the sheath is thought to lead to interference with normal nerve cell function.

Other brain changes associated with age also are linked to memory decline. The grooves on the surface of the brain (sulci) widen. The volume of the ventricles (spaces in the brain that contain cerebrospinal fluid) increases. Blood flow to the brain decreases, as do levels of certain hormones and neurotransmitters that are involved in the transmission of signals among cells in the brain and to and from the brain and other parts of the body.

Twisted protein filaments called neurofibrillary tangles may form inside nerve cells, and clusters of damaged beta-amyloid proteins, called senile plaques, may build up in the brain's gray matter. These are the well-known markers of

Box 2-2: Sharpest seniors have fewer brain tangles linked to AD

A small study may help explain why some older adults stay mentally agile into their 80s and 90s while most older people experience memory decline, according to a March 23, 2010 presentation before the National Meeting of the American Chemical Society. Researchers carefully compared the brains of nine deceased adults over 80 years old who had had no signs of memory decline with the brains of older adults whose memory declined with age. They found that, compared to the brains of people who aged normally, the brains of "super-agers" had many fewer neurofibrillary tangles—twisted fibers of abnormal tau proteins that clutter the brain and In high numbers may damage and eventually kill brain cells. Neurofibrillary tangles are one of the hallmarks of AD. Because most healthy people develop moderate amounts of tangles in their brains as they grow older, scientists had assumed that levels of tau build up gradually in the brain as part of the normal aging process. The new study suggests that tangles influence cognitive performance, and that people with the fewest tangles may perform at superior levels. The scientists plan to focus future research on finding out what makes the cells in the brains of super-agers resistant to tangle formation.

Alzheimer's disease, but they are also present in the brains of older people who show no signs of dementia. A study of the brains of healthy older people whose memories remained exceptionally sharp up to age 80 and beyond revealed that, unlike people who aged normally, these "super-aged" individuals had no neurofibrillary tangles in their brains and appeared to be immune to the formation of the twisted filaments (see Box 2-2).

The effects of age-associated changes become most apparent after age 50, when people may begin to experience an increase in incidents of memory lapse. The older people are, the more difficulty they may have with short-term memory and mental organization. AAMI may cause people to misplace things more easily, occasionally forget a name or phone number, have more trouble multitasking, become easily distracted, or be unable to learn things as easily as they once did.

Mild cognitive impairment (MCI)

The next step in the progression of memory loss—mild cognitive impairment (MCI)—is worse than age-associated memory impairment, but not as serious as dementia (see Chapter 3). People with MCI experience memory difficulties that are beyond those expected for their age group.

"Mild cognitive impairment is a relatively new term, and its definition is in flux," says Deborah Blacker, MD, director of the Gerontology Research Unit at Massachusetts General Hospital. "It's impossible to formulate a precise definition of the disorder because it represents the boundary between normal aging and dementia."

Forgetting things that you would normally remember (such as important appointments), becoming much more reliant on lists and other memory aids, having significantly more trouble remembering what you've just read or seen, or having greater difficulty performing complex tasks (such as cooking a holiday meal) are signs that you may have MCI.

Aside from these issues, people with MCI have normal mental function, can still perform their daily activities, and don't have any symptoms of dementia. Those with MCI are able to follow written or spoken instructions, and can take care of themselves—that is, get dressed by themselves, prepare their meals without assistance, eat their meals, and go on walks without getting lost. In Alzheimer's disease and other dementias, these functions may gradually be lost.

The incidence of mild cognitive impairment in the United States is growing rapidly. It is estimated that the number of cases may be increasing at a rate of up to four percent annually. Currently, as many as 10 to 20 percent of Americans aged 65 and older have MCI, according to the Alzheimer's Association's 2010 Alzheimer's Facts and Figures.

Although MCI is not the same as dementia, research suggests it may increase the risk of developing dementia or Alzheimer's. One analysis of data from 15 studies lasting five years or longer suggests that the rate of progression from MCI to dementia is 4.2 percent annually. The Alzheimer's Association figures are even higher—with as many as 15 percent of people with MCI progressing to dementia each year.

MCI and Alzheimer's share many of the same risk factors, and gender may be an issue as well. Older men are significantly more likely than older women to have mild cognitive impairment. A study of 2,050 randomly selected people between the ages of 70 and 89 living in Minnesota showed that 15 percent of the subjects had MCI, and that men in this age group were one-and-a-half times more likely to have impairment than women. Previous research involving younger seniors has suggested that an equal proportion of men and women develop MCI: This study may indicate that there's a delayed progression of cognitive impairment in men.

Having MCI does not necessarily condemn you to a future in which you can't remember the names of your children and are unable to find your way from the supermarket to your house. Many people with MCI won't progress to dementia, and there are ways to slow the progress of memory loss.

Taking care of your health is crucial to retaining your memory. Get at least 30 minutes of regular aerobic exercise a day to increase the flow of oxygen and nutrients to your brain and boost levels of chemicals that promote cell growth (see Box 2-3) Eat a healthy, low-fat diet with plenty of antioxidant-rich fruits and vegetables, lean meats, fish, low-fat dairy products, legumes and whole grains. Get at least seven hours of sleep a night and manage health conditions—such as cardiovascular problems, high blood pressure and diabetes (see Box 2-4)—that can impair brain function. Keeping your brain active with social interaction, puzzles, and reading helps you resist mental decline. Since recent research suggests that mood symptoms such as agitation and depression increases risk for cognitive decline (see Box 2-5 on the following page), treatment of these symptoms may also slow cognitive decline.

If you believe you or a loved one may have MCI, consult a health care provider who can help determine whether the memory impairment may be associated with a physical or mental disorder that can be treated. Even when no health conditions are identified as causing memory prob-

NEW FINDING

Box 2-3: Vigorous exercise may improve MCI

A preliminary study published in the January 2010 issue of the *Archives of Neurology* found that among a small group of adults with mild cognitive impairment (MCI), those who exercised vigorously for 45 to 60 minutes a day, four days a week, for six months experienced improvements on measures of cognitive function. Participants in the control group—who followed the same schedule but did non-aerobic stretching exercises and kept their heart rates low—did not experience any cognitive improvement. The findings suggest that in addition to providing physical benefits, aerobic exercise that raises the heart rate also provides a cognitive benefit for some adults with MCI.

NEW FINDING

Box 2-4: Diabetes speeds progression of MCI

Prediabetes and diabetes may hasten the decline from mild cognitive impairment to dementia. Scientists followed 963 healthy older adults and 302 older adults with mild cognitive impairment—all 75 years of age and older—for nine years. Over that time period, participants in both groups who had prediabetes (an intermediate stage between normal blood sugar levels and diabetic blood sugar levels) or diabetes had three times the risk of dementia as participants with normal blood sugar, and subjects with MCI. progressed to dementia in 1.83 years, compared with 5 years for participants without blood sugar problems. The research was presented at the July 2010 Alzheimer's Association International Conference on Alzheimer's Disease (ICAD).

Box 2-5: Apathy, agitation, depression linked to faster cognitive decline

Depression, apathy, and agitation may be clinical indicators that a person with MCI will progress to full dementia, according to a study presented July 2010 at ICAD. Researchers assessed neuropsychiatric symptoms in a group of 275 older adults with MCI and tracked their development of dementia over a median of 2.8 years. During that period, study participants with agitation were three times as likely as participants with MCI alone to develop dementia; subjects with apathy were twice as likely to develop dementia, and subjects with depression were 63 percent more likely to develop dementia. Further research is needed to determine whether treating neuropsychiatric symptoms might slow or prevent progression to dementia.

lems, there are medications available that can help improve memory in the early stages of impairment, and improve symptoms such as anxiety or restlessness. Being under a doctor's care also can help ensure that you or your loved one gets optimal care, and that new treatments for memory problems are offered as soon as they become available. Meanwhile, adopting strategies to help in dealing with forgetfulness, such as making lists and keeping calendars of appointments, can help minimize frustration. And because MCI may be a precursor to Alzheimer's in some people, it wouldn't hurt to plan ahead and make decisions regarding future medical care and finances.

When memory impairment becomes more serious

Most people live into their 70s, 80s, and beyond without experiencing memory problems that are more severe than normal age-associated memory impairment. But for some, forgetfulness may get progressively worse and begin to interfere with everyday functioning—important indications that there may be cause for concern. (See Chapter 3 for symptoms of serious memory problems.)

It's important to consult a doctor if you or a loved one seems to be experiencing progressive memory loss. A medical assessment may reveal that the problem is associated with a treatable physical disorder, rather than an irreversible condition such as Alzheimer's disease.

"Understanding normal age-related memory problems and knowing the signs that memory impairment may be getting more serious makes it possible for you to seek early medical intervention if you need it, and to devise coping strategies for your cognitive difficulties," says Dr. Blacker. ∎

3 DEMENTIA

Dementia goes beyond simple forgetfulness; it involves changes in brain function to the point where personality and behavior become affected. According to diagnostic criteria, serious memory lapses may indicate dementia if they are accompanied by at least one other symptom of cognitive decline. Symptoms may include:

- Disorientation with time or place
- Inability to concentrate
- Loss of initiative
- Trouble with executive functions such as planning and organizing
- Language disturbances (aphasia)
- Impaired ability to perform motor activities, without any underlying physical cause (apraxia)
- Problems with spatial reasoning
- Failure to recognize common objects (agnosia)
- Personality and mood changes
- Neglect of personal hygiene and safety.

Primary dementias—such as Alzheimer's disease or dementia with Lewy bodies (DLB)—are characterized by damage to or wasting away of the brain tissue itself, while secondary dementias—such as those associated with depression or thyroid abnormalities—are memory troubles caused by other underlying mental or physical disorders.

Signs of dementia may include asking the same questions over and over; losing the ability to accomplish complex tasks, such as cooking a meal; becoming lost in once-familiar places; forgetting names of familiar people; failing to remember regular appointments; neglecting personal hygiene; showing signs of mental confusion or experiencing mood symptoms such as anxiety, unusual irritability, or depression.

Causes of reversible dementias

Just as with simple memory loss, dementia can be temporarily caused by medical or psychiatric conditions, such as a high fever, vitamin deficiency, head trauma or depression (see Box 3-1). This type of dementia is known as secondary dementia. Because many of the causes of secondary dementia are reversible and can be treated, it's important to see a doctor if you're experiencing sudden memory-loss symptoms, especially if you have had a recent change to your health.

BOX 3-1

Causes of memory loss

Some of the causes of memory loss or forgetfulness, aside from normal aging, include:

- Alzheimer's disease
- Other neurodegenerative diseases such as Parkinson's disease and multiple sclerosis
- Strokes or mini-strokes called transient ischemic attacks (TIAs)
- Head injury or trauma
- Endocrine/metabolic disorders (such as thyroid problems, diabetes, or vitamin B12 deficiency)
- Depression, anxiety or stress
- Normal pressure hydrocephalus (build-up of fluid in the brain)
- Seizures
- General anesthesia
- Alcoholism or substance abuse
- Drugs such as barbiturates, benzodiazepines, sleep medications, painkillers, antihypertensives, heartburn medications, antidepressants, tranquilizers, anxiety medications, antiepileptics, antipsychotics, Parkinson's disease medications, and anticholinergics
- Brain surgery, especially when performed in or near the temporal lobes
- Brain masses caused by tumors or infections
- Herpes encephalitis and other brain infections
- Sleep disorders
- Anoxia (oxygen deprivation) related to heart or lung problems

NEW FINDING

Box-3-2: Analysis calls research on smoking and AD into question

A review by scientists published online in the January 2010 issue of the *Journal of Alzheimer's Disease* provides evidence that smoking is a significant risk factor for Alzheimer's disease (AD)—and reveals that research conducted by people with tobacco company affiliations usually shows the opposite. Researchers reviewed 43 published studies on smoking and AD conducted between 1984 and 2007. After controlling for tobacco industry affiliation of the authors, study design, the quality of the journals in which the research appeared, and the date of publication, the researchers found that industry-affiliated research suggested a reduced risk for AD among smokers, while independent research recorded a near doubling of the risk of AD among smokers. "Our findings point to the ongoing corrosive nature of tobacco Industry funding and point to the need for academic Institutions to decline tobacco Industry funding to protect the research process," said study co-author Stanton A. Glantz, PhD.

The following conditions are among the more common reversible causes of memory loss:

Alcohol and tobacco

Smoking is associated with cognitive decline through effects such as damage to the cardiovascular system that diminishes circulation and increases risk of stroke, and lung abnormalities that may reduce the supply of oxygen to the brain.

Beer, wine and liquor contain ethyl alcohol, a central nervous system depressant that impairs thought processes, motor control and memory, and slows overall brain activity. Going on a drinking binge can leave you with transient amnesia (sometimes referred to as a "blackout"), but chronic alcohol abuse can lead to sometimes-irreversible dementia due to the combined toxic effects of alcohol and the nutritional deficiencies associated with alcoholism (particularly a lack of thiamine—vitamin B1).

Generally, moderate drinking (one or two glasses a day) shouldn't affect your memory. However, if you have a family history of alcohol abuse, you should be especially vigilant and aware of the potentially damaging effects of alcohol on your brain function.

Heavy drinking (more than two alcoholic drinks per day), even without alcohol dependency, can be harmful, recent research shows—especially when combined with heavy smoking (a pack or more of cigarettes a day). In a large study of 938 people over 60 with possible or probable Alzheimer's disease (AD), those who had been smokers or heavy drinkers were quicker to develop symptoms of Alzheimer's disease than people who did neither. Examination of participants' health records showed that subjects who drank more than two drinks a day developed AD 4.8 years sooner than those who drank more moderately. Subjects who smoked more than a pack of cigarettes a day had an onset of AD that was 2.3 years earlier than people who did not smoke as much. Subjects with both risk factors developed the disease five to six years earlier, the authors reported. Both smoking (see Box 3-2) and drinking are thought to harm brain cells and damage communication points between cells known as synapses. The findings suggest that heavy smoking and drinking are important preventable causes of dementia.

Smoking can cause damage to nerve cells in the brain, according to a study published in the June, 2009 issue of the *Journal of Neurochemistry*. Researchers tested the effects of NNK, one of 4,000 chemicals found in cigarettes, on live mice and found that NNK triggered increases in stress-related pro-inflammatory compounds. These substances, in turn, caused white blood cells in the central nervous system to overreact and attack healthy brain cells, causing severe damage to neurons. NNK can enter the body through smoking or chewing tobacco, or through the inhalation of second-hand smoke, the researchers noted.

Fortunately, restricting consumption of alcohol to moderate levels and quitting smoking can benefit brain health no matter what a person's age, according to research reported in the January, 2009 issue of the journal *BMC Geriatrics*. Scientists conducted an analysis of 24 earlier studies exploring the cognitive effects of smoking in older adults. They found that smoking increases risk for Alzheimer's disease among older adults by 79 percent. However, the increased risk was found among those who continued to smoke, not among former smokers, indicating that quitting the habit can be beneficial for the brain at any age.

Inflammation of the brain

Many conditions, particularly meningitis and encephalitis, can lead to a change in mental state. Meningitis affects the meninges, the membranes surrounding the brain and spinal cord. Encephalitis affects the brain tissue itself. Memory loss after one of these illnesses can continue for months or become permanent. Getting prompt treatment is important to help reduce the chance of permanent cognitive loss.

Treatment for both conditions may include antibiotics (often administered intravenously in the hospital) and antiviral agents (depending on cause). Additional treatment for relief of symptoms may include aspirin, acetaminophen, anticonvulsants or corticosteroids.

Systemic infections, too, can lead to thinking and memory impairments (see Box 3-3). Gum disease—gingivitis, a common complaint among older adults— has been linked to lower cognitive performance in some research. In one study researchers analyzed data on more than 7,600 adults ranging in age from 20 to 70 and older to investigate the relationship between gingivitis and mental function. Participants in the study had completed a large national health and nutrition survey and taken mental function tests. The investigators found a significant association between poor oral health (as measured by gum bleeding, loss of attachment of teeth to bone, and tooth loss) and lower performance on cognitive tests. The researchers theorized that one possible cause of the association, which was not influenced by age, might be systemic inflammation linked to periodontal disease.

Depression and anxiety

Major depression is defined as feelings of sadness and hopelessness that last for two weeks or longer. These feelings may be accompanied by other symptoms, such as changes in sleep and appetite, restlessness, fatigue, irritability, and loss of interest in activities previously enjoyed. Cognitive symptoms that mimic the symptoms of dementia, such as confusion, impaired memory, and inability to focus, may affect people with depression.

Long-term depression has a marked effect on the brain: it alters levels of key brain chemicals such as serotonin and norepinephrine, slows activity in the parts of the brain associated with executive function and perception, and shrinks the hippocampus (the part of the brain where memory is processed).

"There's no doubt that depression changes the brain in a number of ways," says Darin Dougherty, MD, MSc, director of the Mood Disorder Section of the Psychiatric Neuroimaging Program at Massachusetts General Hospital. "We don't know as yet whether many of these brain changes are permanent, or whether they will disappear when normal mood is restored, but there is evidence that with exercise, or with therapy, medication or a combination of the two, some of these changes can be reversed."

Long-term anxiety, too, can lead to memory problems. A 12-year study of 1,256 older adults found that people who most often suffered from depression and anxiety were 40 percent more likely to develop mild cognitive impairment than people who were least apt to suffer from these negative states.

Depression is typically treated with medications such as selective serotonin reuptake inhibitors (SSRIs), and/or psychotherapy. Anxiety is treated with relaxation therapy, psychotherapy, and/or medications such as anti-anxiety drugs, antidepressants, and beta-blockers.

Drug effects and interactions

Certain classes of prescription and over-the-counter drugs are known to affect memory and brain function. These include antidepressants, sleeping pills, anti-anxiety medications, painkillers, and some antihistamines.

Cancer patients can develop memory loss or confusion during their treatment. Cognitive deficits related to chemotherapy—sometimes called "chemo brain"—may occur in most patients who receive either chemotherapy or radiation, according to one study. Investigators tested 595 patients, most of whom were being treated with chemotherapy, with or without radiation, for breast or prostate cancers. The participants self-rated their problems with memory and concentration before treatment began, immediately after treatment concluded, and at six months after treatment. The majority of participants who were undergoing chemotherapy and radiation reported experiencing memory loss and difficulty concentrating. The problems worsened during treatment, and persisted for at least six months after treatment ended.

Other research suggests that the cognitive effects caused by one commonly used chemotherapy drug may result from damage to the cells of the central nervous system.

The chemotherapy drug 5-fluorouracil (5-FU), which is used to treat cancers of the breast, ovaries, colon, stomach, and elsewhere, causes cognitive symptoms that worsen with time, and continue after treatment is ended, according to a study published in the April 22, 2008 *Journal of Biology*. The study, which involved research with laboratory animals, suggests a possible explanation for symptoms of memory loss and trouble concentrating that affects up to 50 percent of patients treated with 5-FU. Examination of mice exposed to 5-FU revealed that the drug damaged progenitor cells—basic cells in the central nervous system that later mature into various specialized cells.

Researchers also found evidence that the drug injured cells that produce a fatty substance called myelin, which coats nerve cells and helps them communicate with one another. Cell injury appears to progress over time, with damage far worse after six months than a week after treatment, the researchers reported. The study offers the first possible explanation for "chemo brain," and may help scientists find a way to decrease or eliminate cell damage caused by the cancer drug, along with accompanying cognitive symptoms.

Anticholinergic drugs, commonly used to treat disorders such as ulcers, stomach cramps, Parkinson's disease, urinary incontinence, insomnia and motion sickness, also can lead to declines in thinking skills in healthy older adults, according to one long-term study. Researchers assessed the cognitive performance of 870 men and women with an average age of 75 once a year for eight years, comparing the thinking skills of subjects who took at least one anticholinergic medication with those who took none. They found that among participants taking anticholinergic medications, the rate of decline in memory and other cognitive functions was 1.5 times faster than the rate in people who were not taking the medications; among those taking the drugs for Parkinson's disease and bladder problems the rate of decline was three times faster. Changes associated with the drugs amounted to a "small slippage" over a period of years, however, and the drugs were not associated with an increased risk for Alzheimer's disease, the study authors noted.

Even cholesterol-lowering statin drugs—valued for their ability to lower risk of cardiovascular disease—have been associated with cognitive impairment in some individuals. Anecdotal information suggests that some people who use the drugs experience memory problems, and recent research has offered a plausible explanation for these brain effects. Statins may adversely affect the brain by blocking the production of cholesterol needed for optimal cognitive functioning, according to a study published in the February 2009 issue of *Proceedings of the National Academy of Sciences*. Cholesterol produced within the brain encourages brain cells to release neurotransmitters, chemicals that help transmit signals from cell to cell and make information processing and memory possible. Statins are designed to attack the machinery of cholesterol synthesis in the liver, but the medication also goes to the brain, where it reduces the synthesis of cholesterol necessary to that organ. Working with brain cells in a laboratory setting, investigators measured the release of neurotransmitters by the cells in the presence of cholesterol and in the absence of the fatty substance. They found that the cells released five times the quantity of neurotransmitters when cholesterol was present. The authors cautioned that for many people, taking statins can be very healthful and urged statin users to consult with their doctors about the medication. Eating cholesterol-laden foods will not affect brain function, since cholesterol in the blood cannot cross the blood-brain barrier. Fortunately, memory complaints associated with statins can often be addressed effectively by lowering the dosage or changing the type of statin prescribed.

If you are experiencing memory problems—and especially if you recently began taking a new medication or switched to a higher dosage of an existing medication—ask your doctor whether any of the medications you're taking might affect your memory. Drug-related memory impairment usually can be resolved by switching medications, changing dosage levels or stopping the drug entirely.

Lung problems

Keeping your lungs healthy and functioning at optimal capacity is important to your brain, studies suggest. Treating conditions that impair respiratory functioning—including allergic rhinitis, commonly known as hay fever—can help improve memory performance. In some cases, treatment may also lower long-term risk of more serious memory impairment.

Cognitive functions such as attention and memory that require sustained mental effort may be impaired by allergic rhinitis (often called hay fever), according to a study published February 18, 2009 in the online edition of *Clinical & Experimental Allergy*. Researchers asked 25 volunteers who had seasonal allergic rhinitis and 26 comparable healthy controls to complete a battery of demanding cognitive tests of various lengths and to respond to subjective questionnaires. All participants were tested before exposure to allergens, and again following exposure to allergens. The tests were designed to measure cognitive functions such as sustained attention, short- and long-term memory and speed of information processing. Researchers also used visual rating scales to assess the amount of mental effort expended by participants in completing tasks.

The investigation revealed that both groups of participants did well on short tasks, but compared to participants without allergies, subjects who had allergic rhinitis experienced a significant decline in cognitive performance when tackling the longer mental tasks. The allergic participants were able to compensate for cognitive problems on short tasks by expending additional effort, but during sustained tasks of longer duration they responded more slowly and made more errors than the healthy participants, the researchers said.

In one investigation, researchers from the University of Washington in Seattle found a statistically significant correlation between poor lung function and an increased risk of developing dementia. The scientists tested lung function in 2,418 people age 65 or older, using lung spirometry studies to assess how well they were able to inhale and exhale air. Over a six-year period, participants who did poorly on the spirometry tests were more likely to develop dementia, according to the research team. Those who scored in the lowest quartile on the lung capacity test had nearly three times the risk of dementia compared to those who scored the highest. Although the study didn't conclude that poor lung health caused dementia, it suggested that maintaining good lung function by preventing and treating lung diseases might decrease dementia risk in older adults.

Metabolic disease or abnormalities

Certain metabolic diseases, such as diabetes, liver or kidney failure, and thyroid disease can wreak havoc on your memory, researchers have found. Research suggests that cognitive impairment can result from increased or decreased concentrations of thyroid hormones, especially in older people. Clinical and subclinical hypothyroidism (decreased thyroid function) as well as hyperthyroidism (overactive thyroid function) in middle-aged and elderly adults have been linked with impairment of memory, visuospatial organization, attention, and reaction time. Even subtle variations in thyroid function can cause significant cognitive effects. Moreover, decreased thyroid function can lead to mood states such as depression or apathy that may be mistaken for symptoms of dementia.

A 12-year study of older adults suggests that over the long term, untreated thyroid dysfunction may lead to higher rates of dementia as well. In the study, which was reported in the July 28, 2008 issue of the *Archives of Internal Medicine*, women who had unusually high or low levels of the thyroid hormone thyrotropin had more than twice the risk of developing AD as women with normal levels. Fortunately, thyroid problems can be detected through a simple blood test and effective treatment is available that can restore thyroid hormones to normal levels in most cases.

Diabetes mellitus – a disease characterized by the body's inability to use glucose (sugar) properly – can also cause cognitive symptoms that may be mistaken for dementia. Both type 1 diabetes (caused by a failure of the pancreas to produce sufficient quantities of insulin that enables cells to metabolize sugar) and type 2 diabetes (in which the body loses its sensitivity to the actions of insulin) interfere with the absorption of sugar from the bloodstream into body cells. Insufficient glucose

Box 3-4: Diabetes trebles risk of dementia among people with MCI

Researchers have found that individuals with diabetes who have mild cognitive impairment (MCI, memory loss that is greater than normal for an individual's age group, but does not meet the criteria for dementia) are at much greater risk of progressing to dementia than individuals who have MCI, but do not have diabetes. In a four-year study of that followed 103 men and women over age 65 with MCI, researchers found that the 16 participants with diabetes had nearly three times the risk of developing dementia as participants without diabetes, according to a report in the January 2010 issue of *The British Journal of Psychiatry*. After adjusting for socio-demographic and genetic background, medical conditions, and other factors, only diabetes was associated with progression to dementia, the researchers said.

in the bloodstream, called hypoglycemia, can cause people to feel light-headed or confused, or to have difficulty speaking. Long-term hyperglycemia, in which blood glucose levels remain higher than normal for two months or more, can cause impaired thinking, according to a recent study.

Researchers tracked blood glucose levels in about 3,000 older adults (average age 63) with type 2 diabetes over two to three months. They also measured participants' intellectual performance in a series of four 30-minute tests assessing memory, visual motor speed, and capacity for learning and managing multiple tasks. The investigators found that participants with chronically high blood sugar levels fared worse on cognitive tests than those with lower blood sugar levels. Although the study did not prove that lowering blood sugar can slow the rate of cognitive decline in a person with diabetes, the results add to a growing body of evidence that suggests uncontrolled blood glucose levels may speed cognitive aging among people with diabetes.

Research suggests that, overall, people who have diabetes are at increased risk for dementia (see Box 3-4). Although researchers don't know exactly why this is the case, they speculate that it may be because diabetes plays a role in hardening and narrowing of blood vessels (atherosclerosis), which can reduce or block blood flow to brain tissue and deprive brain cells of necessary oxygen and nutrients. Depending on where the blockage in the blood vessel occurs, memory can be affected. Some studies suggest that diabetes may be associated with brain atrophy in the brain's frontal lobes (responsible for attention and long-term memory, among other functions) and temporal lobes (responsible for language skills and memory of verbal and non-verbal information, among other functions). Other research suggests that beta-amyloid, a protein that builds up in the brains of people with Alzheimer's disease, also forms in the pancreas of people with type 2 diabetes, indicating that the same underlying factors may lead to both conditions.

People with metabolic syndrome, characterized by a cluster of risk factors such as abdominal obesity, elevated cholesterol and high blood pressure, as well as type 2 diabetes often have insulin resistance, in which their body no longer responds appropriately to the release of insulin from the pancreas. As a result, glucose doesn't leave the blood and enter the cells as it should, so the pancreas produces more insulin to compensate. This excess insulin can lead to inflammation and damage to the brain.

Excess belly fat associated with metabolic syndrome (having an apple shape as opposed to a pear shape) has been linked to increased risk of Alzheimer's disease. Investigators looked at the medical records of 6,583 members of a health-care plan whose belly fat was measured when they were 40 to 45 years old, and who were then followed-up to see who had developed Alzheimer's or other dementia an average of 36 years later, when they were in their 70s and 80s. Their findings:

Obese study participants with the highest levels of belly fat in their 40s were 3.6 times more likely to develop dementia in old age than obese subjects who had the least amount of belly fat. Overweight subjects with the greatest amount of abdominal fat in mid-life were 2.3 times more likely to develop dementia as seniors than overweight participants with the lowest levels of belly fat. Normal-weight subjects with high belly fat were 89 percent more likely to have dementia later on than people of normal weight who had little belly fat in their 40s.

Although the study does not prove that belly fat causes dementia, it implies an association between high levels of fat in the abdomen and negative effects on the brain. The study's authors theorized that these effects may be related to toxins and hormones secreted by abdominal fat, and urged people with high amounts of belly fat to lose weight to reduce their risk.

Keeping diabetes under control can help prevent many complications of the disease, including memory problems. Managing diabetes involves eating a healthy diet, exercising, carefully monitoring blood sugar levels, and taking diabetes medications, if necessary. Losing weight, and especially belly fat, also may help avoid harm to your memory.

Normal pressure hydrocephalus

A condition called normal pressure hydrocephalus (NPH) occurs when cerebrospinal fluid builds up in the ventricles, or cavities, of the brain, causing increased pressure on fragile brain tissue that may lead to impairment or dementia. It's most common in older adults, but also can be caused by head trauma, tumor or infection. If caught early, NPH can be treated by draining excess fluid from the brain. Without treatment, it can lead to dementia.

Sleep problems

Most people require at least six hours of sleep each night in order for their memory to perform at its peak. With age, it's common to have greater difficulty falling or staying asleep, often because of underlying problems such as arthritis, pain, depression or frequent urination. Since research shows a direct link between sleep deprivation and memory loss, optimizing sleep time will not only make you feel more rested, but also less forgetful and better able to cope with stress. Getting a good night's sleep also might help improve your ability to retain new information.

Harvard researchers asked 48 young, healthy volunteers to learn a group of 20 word pairs—such as baseball/window. However, the way in which the participants were tested on the different word groups differed. Two groups were taught the words at 9 a.m. and were tested at 9 p.m. the same day. Two other groups learned

Box 3-5: Severe sleep apnea may cause brain damage

Researchers have discovered evidence that severe obstructive sleep apnea (OSA)—a disorder characterized by repeated cessation of breathing for short periods during sleep—may cause deficits in concentrations of gray matter in several areas of the brain. Researchers compared brain scans of 36 men with OSA to brain scans of 31 healthy, age-matched peers looking for structural differences in gray matter, the part of the brain where the majority of information processing takes place. The scientists found that compared to healthy subjects, the subjects with OSA had lower concentrations of gray matter in the prefrontal cortex, cerebellum, and other regions, according to a report published in the February 1, 2010 issue of the journal *Sleep*. The structural changes may help explain the higher risk for cognitive problems such as memory impairment and executive dysfunction, emotional problems, abnormalities in cardiovascular function, and dysfunctions of autonomic and respiratory control experienced by individuals with OSA. The study authors recommended that people with OSA seek therapy with continuous positive airway pressure to stop further injury to their brains.

the words at 9 p.m. and were tested the following morning at 9 a.m., after a night's sleep. One of each of the two groups was taught a second set of words to see if it would interfere with their memory of the first word set. Researchers found that people who tried to remember word pairs after sleeping overnight had greater recall, even with interference, suggesting that sleep not only aids in remembering, but also helps solidify memories.

Sleep disorders that may be tied to memory problems include sleep apnea—a condition often linked to obesity that causes people to stop breathing repeatedly during the night. The brain continually jolts the body awake to restart breathing. People with sleep apnea may be unaware that they are waking up, but will feel tired the next day. Daytime napping, which is thought to be a consequence of sleep apnea, has been linked in one study to greater risk for brain-injuring stroke, which also can damage memory. Older adults who reported "some" dozing during the day were more than twice as likely to suffer a stroke than people who reported no napping, and adults who reported nodding off frequently were more than four times as likely to experience a stroke.

A nine-year study of 5,422 men and women published in the March 25, 2010 online edition of the *American Journal of Respiratory and Critical Care* found that risk for stroke rose with the severity of sleep apnea in middle-age and older men, with severe sleep apnea linked to three times normal risk. Increased risk in women was significantly associated with severe levels of sleep apnea, the researchers found.

The increased risk of stroke associated with untreated sleep apnea may reflect the wear and tear on the brain caused by fluctuations in blood pressure, according to another study. Researchers who compared 22 middle-aged adults with untreated sleep apnea to a control group of 26 adults without apnea, measuring subjects' blood pressure as they slept and testing changes in blood pressure as they squatted and then stood up suddenly. They found that as blood pressure within cerebral blood vessels rose, sleep apnea subjects experienced a drop in blood flow to the brain, suggesting they did not compensate as well for blood pressure changes as people without apnea. The researchers theorized that the recurring rise and fall of blood pressure associated with sleep apnea gradually erodes the brain's ability to compensate for blood pressure changes and creates an increasing susceptibility to stroke. They urged early diagnosis and treatment for sleep apnea to prevent damage to the brain.

More evidence that treatment for sleep apnea is essential to protect the brain was provided by research published recently in the journal *Sleep* (see Box 3-5). Continuous positive airway pressure (CPAP), which forces air into the lungs via a special machine, can help many of those with obstructive sleep apnea get a good night's sleep.

Another sleep disorder called restless legs syndrome (RLS) interferes with sleep by causing unpleasant sensations in the legs that occur just before falling asleep, or during the night. Today there are medications that may be helpful for RLS.

You can treat many sleep problems by practicing good sleep "hygiene" (such as going to bed and waking up at the same time each day; avoiding caffeine and alcohol before bed; exercising regularly—but not before bedtime; and using your bed only for sleep or sex). If you seek medical help for a sleep problem, your doctor will attempt to find the cause of your sleep problem and may prescribe appropriate medication. Rarely are "sleeping pills" required and, if prescribed, they should be taken only for a short period of time. As noted previously, they can sometimes worsen memory.

Stress

Research has found that major life stressors, such as going through a financial reversal, experiencing a catastrophic accident, or losing a loved one, can impair memory function and contribute to memory loss. An excess of stress hormones released in response to stressors can damage the brain cells involved in memory.

Learning how to manage your stress and anxiety is important to keeping your memory functioning at its peak. Protect your memory by taking measures to reduce or avoid stressful situations, using relaxation techniques (such as meditation or soothing music) or exercise to reduce the impact of stress, or seeking mental-health counseling to help you deal with profound or chronic stressors in your life.

Vitamin deficiency

Pernicious anemia caused by an inability to absorb vitamin B-12 also can cause cognitive changes that mimic the symptoms of dementia. Vitamin B12 is essential for the brain to function properly. A lack of this vitamin can permanently damage brain cells. As you age, your rate of nutrient absorption slows, making it more difficult for your system to get the essential vitamins that it requires. If you drink alcohol or smoke, you are at an even greater risk of having vitamin deficiencies because both leach nutrients from the body.

Symptoms of vitamin B12 deficiency include: anemia; loss of appetite; fatigue; constipation; numbness and tingling of hands and feet; shortness of breath; weakness; sore mouth and tongue; weight loss; difficulty maintaining balance; depression; poor memory; and confusion.

Vitamin B12 deficiency can be treated via a monthly injection. If you are B12-deficient, addressing the issue early can help you recover some, if not all, lost memory function. Without treatment, a vitamin B12 deficiency can lead to increasing memory loss and progressive nerve damage.

Memory loss also might occur with a vitamin B1 deficiency following gastric bypass surgery for obesity, research suggests. In rare cases, people who experience severe vomiting after the surgery can develop a complication called Wernicke encephalopathy, in which they are deficient in vitamin B1 (thiamine). This condition can lead to memory loss, as well as coordination and vision problems. Wernicke encephalopathy can be reversed with intravenous infusions of vitamin B1, but it's important to seek treatment for this condition as quickly as possible to ensure a full recovery.

Vitamin D deficiency may also harm brain function, according to a recent study. Researchers analyzing data from a large population-based health survey have found that among 1,766 adults ages 65 and older, low blood levels of vitamin D were significantly associated with cognitive impairment. The study, published in the February 2009 issue of the *Journal of Geriatric Psychology and Neurology*, Subjects who had the lowest levels of vitamin D were more than twice as likely as those with the highest levels to show signs of cognitive impairment in mental tests that assessed attention, orientation in time and space and memory, the researchers found. The study authors recommended further research to discover whether supplementation with vitamin D could reduce the incidence of cognitive impairment.

A more recent large study provides additional evidence that vitamin D deficiency increases the risk for cognitive impairment in older women (see Box 3-6).

Causes of irreversible dementia

Other types of dementia are caused by progressive brain damage, and are irreversible. These are known as primary dementias. The most commonly known form of irreversible dementia is Alzheimer's disease, which is discussed in greater detail in Chapter 4. The following are other causes of progressive dementia:

Dementia with Lewy bodies (DLB)

Dementia with Lewy bodies (DLB) is believed to be one of the most common forms of primary dementia, second only to Alzheimer's disease. DLB is caused by the build-up of proteins called Lewy bodies inside neurons in the part of the brain responsible for memory, language and consciousness. It's thought to be related to Parkinson's disease, and people who have it often develop Parkinson's-like muscle rigidity. Other symptoms include drowsiness, lethargy, slurred speech, sleep abnormalities, irritability, agitation and hallucinations. Although no cure exists for DLB, medication can help control the cognitive symptoms. The main drugs used to treat the cognitive symptoms of DLB are acetylcholinesterase inhibitors such as donepezil (Aricept) and rivastigmine (Exelon).

Fronto-temporal dementias (FTD)

This relatively rare spectrum of disorders causes parts of the frontal and temporal lobes of the brain, which control memory, personality and language skills, to slowly atrophy. FTD is most common in people younger than 65. Symptoms tend to come on slowly, and typically involve inappropriate behavior, difficulty finding the right words, and personality changes. In its late stages, FTD resembles Alzheimer's disease, with significant memory impairment. Although no treatment for FTD exists, various classes of psychiatric medications may help control the behavioral symptoms.

Parkinson's disease (PD)

Parkinson's disease (PD) is a chronic and progressive disease of the nervous system. It occurs when brain cells that produce the chemical dopamine die. Because dopamine is essential for normal movement, people with Parkinson's develop muscle rigidity in the limbs, as well as tremors and balance difficulties. Parkinson's also affects cognitive function, leading to depression, hallucinations and anxiety. An estimated 20 percent of people with Parkinson's disease will develop dementia, usually after age 70. Mild Parkinsonian signs, such as muscle rigidity and tremors, are associated with increased risk of dementia, according to a recent study (see Box 3-7).

Research suggests that the earlier people with PD develop dementia the shorter their survival times may be. A 12-year study of 233 patients with Parkinson's disease (PD) conducted by researchers in Norway revealed that men who already had dementia by the time they reached age 70 had a life expectancy of 4.2 years, while women who had dementia at 70 could expect to live 5.7 years. Among participants who had no dementia on their 70th birthdays, men had a life expectancy of eight years, of which five would be dementia-free, and women had a life expectancy of 11 years, seven of which would be dementia-free. The researchers also found that the incidence of dementia steadily grew with increased age and duration of Parkinson's disease, so that by age 90, between 80 and 90 percent of participants had dementia.

Cognitive problems characteristic of Parkinson's can be treated with cholinesterase inhibitors—the medication Rivastigmine (Exelon) has been approved by the FDA for this form of dementia. Overall, Parkinson's is treated with medications that are either precursors to dopamine (levodopa and carbidopa), or drugs that replicate the natural effects of dopamine (bromocriptine, apomorphine, pramipexole, and ropinirole). Anticholinergic drugs are also used. However, all of these drugs potentially can cause cognitive, mood, and thought disorders (i.e. hallucinations and delusions).

Another medication, memantine (Namenda), an N-methyl-D-aspartate (NMDA)–receptor antagonist that is already approved for use in moderate to severe AD, may be effective against Parkinson's disease as well. In an early trial, the drug was associated with a small, but significant change for the better in study participants with Parkinson's disease the drug compared to participants who received placebo, according to a report published in the July 2009 issue of *Lancet Neurology*. Results of a larger trial are expected soon.

Cardiovascular disease

As many as 25 percent of cases of severe memory loss are triggered by strokes that destroy cells in regions of the brain that are involved in learning and memory. Major strokes involve the rupture or blockage of blood vessels in the brain, causing cell injury or death by interrupting blood flow and starving brain cells of oxygen and nutrients (see Box 3-8). Atrial fibrillation (A-fib), a common condition characterized by irregular heartbeat, also increases risk for AD and other forms of dementia. In atrial fibrillation, chaotic pumping actions of the upper chambers of the heart cause blood to pool and raise the risk of blood clots that can lead to stroke. One in 20 people over 65, and one in 10 over 80 has A-fib, which more than doubles the risk of AD, but a recent study shows risk can be lowered through use of a treatment called catheter ablation (see Box 3-9).

NEW FINDING

Box 3-9: Treatment that cures heart arrhythmia appears to lower Alzheimer's risk

Using a procedure called catheter ablation to treat a common heart arrhythmia may be a highly effective way of lowering risk for Alzheimer's disease (AD) and other forms of dementia, brain-damaging stroke, and overall mortality, a new study suggests. The technique is one of two common treatments for atrial fibrillation or A-fib, in which irregular pumping actions of the upper chambers of the heart cause blood to pool and raise the risk of blood clots. One in 20 people over 65, and one in 10 over 80 has A-fib, which more than doubles the risk of AD. In catheter ablation, a catheter is threaded through veins in the legs up to the heart, where abnormal heart tissue is cauterized, eliminating irregular heartbeats and curing A-fib in about 64 percent of cases. Researchers compared long-term outcomes in about 4,200 people who received catheter ablation with outcomes in 16,800 people who were treated with medication, another common therapy. The scientists followed participants for three years, and found that 0.2 percent of people who underwent ablation developed AD, compared to 0.9 percent of people treated with medication. Approximately 0.4 percent of people treated with ablation developed other types of dementia, compared to 1.9 percent of people treated with medications; 2.2 percent of people who underwent ablation had a stroke compared to 4.7 percent of participants who received medications; and approximately 6 percent of participants who underwent ablation died, compared to 23.5 percent of participants who took medications. The findings were presented May 13, 2010 at the annual scientific meeting of the Heart Rhythm Society.

A slower, stepwise process of injury to brain cells may occur as the result of a series of transient ischemic attacks (TIAs, or "mini-strokes") that affect small areas of brain cells but may have a damaging cumulative effect, or by disease of the small blood vessels of the brain. The condition that results from these various vascular events is called vascular dementia (VaD), and it can involve permanent damage to the brain.

Disruption of blood flow to the brain can lead to extensive tissue damage. Major strokes affecting larger areas of the brain are associated with the sudden onset of symptoms that may involve significant impairment in cognition, depending on the area of the brain that is affected. With multiple small strokes, symptoms usually appear gradually as the damage spreads, and can include memory loss, shuffling movements, inappropriate behavior, and loss of bladder or bowel control.

Strokes may occur without recognizable symptoms (transient ischemic attacks, or "silent strokes"), and these events, too can cause brain damage and increase the chances that an individual may suffer a more devastating stroke in the future. A new study suggests that many apparently healthy older adults have unknowingly suffered at least one silent stroke with brain injury (see Box 3-10). This startling finding underscores the widespread dangers of stroke and the importance of lowering cardiovascular risk factors such as hypertension and high cholesterol that can lead to blockage or hemorrhage of a blood vessel in the brain, experts say.

Although it's not possible to reverse the damage caused by a stroke or other

NEW FINDING

Box 3-10: Most people unaware they've suffered a "silent stroke"

Researchers found reason to worry about stroke awareness in the general public after analyzing data on 1,000 men and women with an average age of 73 who had suffered a minor stroke or transient ischemic attack (TIA, often called a "silent stroke"). They found that 69 percent of the minor stroke patients they studied and 68 percent of the TIA patients did not understand what had caused their symptoms, and that only 46 and 47 percent, respectively, had sought treatment within the three-hour window for use of a clot-busting drug that minimizes brain damage. Although the majority of patients sought medical care within 24 hours, 77 percent went to their physicians first rather than to an emergency care facility, where they would have received more rapid attention, according to a report on the study in the April 15, 2010 issue of the journal *Stroke*. Both TIA and minor stroke occur when a blood vessel is temporarily clogged, blocking blood flow to the brain. The study's findings suggest that much of the public is still unaware of the symptoms that indicate TIA or stroke, such as difficulty speaking or temporary weakness or numbness of an arm or leg. Although TIA and minor strokes usually do not cause permanent damage, they are considered a medical emergency that requires prompt attention to reduce risk of a subsequent, more serious, stroke.

Box 3-11: Exposure to pesticides can boost risk of Alzheimer's

Researchers recruited adults 65 years of age and older who lived in Cache County, Utah, and asked them to complete detailed occupational history questionnaires that included information about exposure to various types of pesticides. The cognitive status of participants was assessed at the outset of the study, and again after three, seven and ten years. Researchers also recorded the diagnosis of dementia and AD to evaluate the risk of incident dementia and AD associated with pesticide exposure. According to a report published in the May 11, 2010 issue of *Neurology*, exposure to pesticides significantly increased the risk for all-cause dementia. The risk of AD associated with exposure to organophosphates was slightly higher than the risk associated with organochlorines, the researchers found.

forms of VaD, it may be possible to avoid further injury to brain cells through simple lifestyle changes. Since cardiovascular disease is a major risk factor for stroke, controlling blood pressure and cholesterol, losing weight, quitting smoking, and managing conditions such as diabetes, atrial fibrillation, and coronary artery disease can reduce the risk of vascular events that may cause further impairment. Eating a nutritious, low-fat diet and exercising regularly also can help.

Researchers are looking at whether dementia drugs such as memantine (Namenda), donepezil (Aricept), galantamine (Razadyne) and rivastigmine (Exelon) might be effective for VaD.

Exposure to toxins

Researchers have found evidence of a connection between exposure to environmental toxins such as pesticides and greater risk for dementia and Alzheimer's disease later in life (see Box 3-11). One study found that older individuals who had lived in cities with severe air pollution before they died showed more evidence of brain inflammation and accumulation of beta-amyloid upon brain autopsy than comparable older people who lived in unpolluted areas. Researchers have also found that older adults with high levels of lead in their bodies scored lower on tests of cognition than people who had not accumulated excess levels of the toxic metal.

Chronic inflammation

Chronic inflammation caused by an immune system gone haywire has also been implicated in the development of Alzheimer's disease. A team of researchers at Massachusetts General Hospital has found evidence that factors that trigger hyperactivity of the innate immune system—not only infection, but also traumatic brain injury and stroke, which are already known to increase the risk for Alzheimer's—could initiate a process of excessive deposition of beta-amyloid that leads to AD (see Box 3-12).

The warning signs

Occasional trouble recalling names, or forgetting an appointment from time to time are not signs that you have dementia. But trouble remembering how to do things you've done many times before, getting to a place you've been to often, or planning a complicated meal should raise concerns. Other signs of a serious memory problem are asking people to repeat themselves many times, having significantly more trouble learning new skills than you used to, or difficulty with simple transactions (for example, paying for food at the supermarket).

"It's not just occasional forgetting, it's memory loss that affects other areas of functioning and it's impairing," says William Falk, MD, director of Outpatient Geriatric Psychiatry at Massachusetts General Hospital. "You may have difficulty remembering what to call many things, or forget the names of people close to you. You may fail to recognize familiar objects or people. You may find complex tasks impossible to accomplish. Things you used to do before you can't do now. Often other people may notice your memory problems before you do. At this point, other contributing factors must be ruled out. You must be evaluated by a doctor."

Anyone who has dementia should be under the care of a family doctor, internist, neurologist, psychiatrist or geriatrician. A doctor should be able to determine whether your memory problems are caused by treatable conditions, such as the side effects of medicine, thyroid problems or a bout of depression. Even if the doctor diagnoses an irreversible form of dementia, it is possible to treat the physical and behavioral problems associated with the condition, and to get help in coping with it. ■

Box 3-12: MGH study: Protein associated with AD may be part of the immune system

Beta-amyloid proteins—which are toxic to brain cells and a primary constituent of brain plaques associated with Alzheimer's disease (AD)—may actually be part of the body's natural immune defenses. Research conducted at MGH and published in the March 3, 2010 *PLosOne* suggests the proteins act as effective antimicrobial agents against a variety of pathogens in the brain until unknown factors trigger their accumulation into brain-clogging plaques. Understanding the normal function of beta-amyloid might lead to promising new therapies against the Alzheimer's.

Researchers looked into similarities between beta-amyloid proteins and antimicrobial peptides, small proteins that cross the blood-brain barrier to fight infection within the central nervous system and brain. The investigators compared the antimicrobial activity of synthetic versions of beta-amyloid proteins with the activity of an antimicrobial peptide known as LL-37, with which beta-amyloid proteins share a number of similar physical, chemical and biological traits. The researchers found that beta-amyloid proteins were able to inhibit growth in eight of 15 pathogens tested, and were as strong as or stronger than LL-37 against seven of those pathogens. They then tested brain tissue containing high levels of beta-amyloid from AD patients to determine whether antimicrobial activity would be produced by Alzheimer's-associated beta-amyloid and found that—compared to brain tissue from age-matched controls that had no antimicrobial effects—tissue from AD patients had significant antimicrobial activity.

The researchers believe that chronic activation of the immune system in response to an infection of the central nervous system—or to known AD risk factors such as stroke or head injury—might trigger excessive production and accumulation of beta-amyloid and lead to a destructive inflammatory response within the brain. Determining what factors trigger the innate immune system and cause the accumulation of beta-amyloid may lead to ways to prevent or control that response.

4 ALZHEIMER'S DISEASE

More than five million Americans are coping with Alzheimer's disease (AD), according to data released by the Alzheimer's Association, and the numbers are rising. The disease is a "looming global epidemic," with 107 million Alzheimer's patients expected worldwide by the year 2050, say researchers from the Johns Hopkins Bloomberg School of Public Health.

Alzheimer's disease is the most common cause of dementia, accounting for more than 50 percent of all cases in people age 65 and older. Although Alzheimer's usually begins after age 60, it can very rarely affect people as young as 30.

Alzheimer's disease damages the brain's intellectual functions—memory, orientation and thinking. Memory gradually deteriorates, impairing the person's judgment and affecting his or her ability to perform normal daily activities.

The brain relies on nerve cells called neurons to process information. In people with Alzheimer's, these neurons become damaged to the point where normal functioning is impaired. The two primary hallmarks of AD are plaques and neurofibrillary tangles. Plaques are formed by sticky clusters of a protein called beta-amyloid, which accumulate between nerve cells. Tangles are twisted clumps of another protein, called tau (see Box 4-1); abnormal accumulations of tau develop within the neurons themselves as part of the disease process.

Researchers believe that plaques and tangles disrupt normal brain cell activity, and block the transmission of signals between neurons, essentially shutting down communication in parts of the brain. But whether they are a primary cause of AD, or symptoms of an underlying disease mechanism, is not yet clear.

BOX 4-1: NORMAL BRAIN NEURONS VS. ALZHEIMER'S BRAIN NEURONS

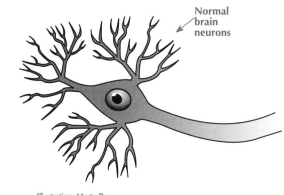

Normal brain neurons

Illustration: Marty Bee

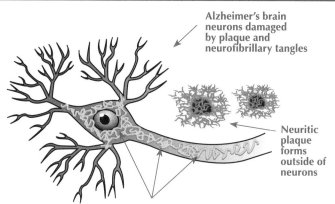

Alzheimer's brain neurons damaged by plaque and neurofibrillary tangles

Neuritic plaque forms outside of neurons

Neurofibrillary tangles are formed inside the neurons by twisted clumps of the protein "tau"

The stages of Alzheimer's

People who have Alzheimer's typically go through a series of stages, in which symptoms gradually worsen (see Box 4-2). However, not everyone will go through all of these stages or progress at the same rate:

■ **Mild cognitive impairment.** Although MCI is technically not a stage of Alzheimer's disease, and may not progress to AD, most people who develop the memory disorder will experience this stage of memory loss. The person with MCI will have significantly more trouble remembering simple things—for example, a familiar telephone number, or where he or she put the car keys. The person will start to have more trouble remembering names or words, performing complex tasks, and acquiring and retaining information. These memory lapses may become increasingly noticeable to others.

■ **Early-stage Alzheimer's.** As the condition progresses, it becomes more difficult to handle multi-step tasks, such as making dinner with several courses or setting up a filing system for household bills. The person might seem increasingly withdrawn in social situations, or have trouble recalling current or historical events. Psychological problems, such as personality changes, irritability, anxiety or depression, may emerge at this stage, putting strain on the individual's relationships with family and friends.

■ **Mid-stage Alzheimer's.** Assisted care usually becomes necessary at this stage. The person will be unable to remember important information, such as his or her address or phone number. He or she will need help picking out clothes and remembering the date and time. The person may become delusional at times and express irrational fears—for example, that someone is stealing from him or her.

BOX 4-2: THE STAGES OF ALZHEIMER'S

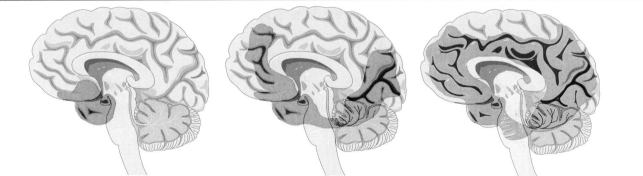

Alzheimer's disease (AD) seems to begin in a small area of the brain called the entorhinal cortex (left). Plaques and tangles then spread to the hippocampus (middle), where short- and long-term memories are formed. As AD progresses from moderate to severe, damage spreads (right) to areas that affect language, reasoning, sensory processing and thought, until plaques and tangles are widespread in the brain. Illustration from *Mind Mood & Memory.*

■ Moderately severe and late-stage Alzheimer's. Cognitive ability becomes seriously compromised at this stage. The person will need help performing even the simplest tasks, such as using the bathroom or eating. By late-stage Alzheimer's, the ability to recognize one's loved ones is lost. The person will become unable to communicate, walk without assistance, or react to his or her environment.

Although scientists are making progress in understanding Alzheimer's disease, no cure for the condition has been found. Medications may help slow its progress, but at this date the disease is irreversible. However, treatments and support systems can significantly improve quality of life for people with the disease.

Risks for Alzheimer's

The overall risk for developing Alzheimer's is 10 to 15 percent, but several factors can increase your odds of developing the disease:

Age

The single biggest risk for Alzheimer's disease is increasing age. After you reach age 65, your risk doubles about every five years. By age 85, about half of all people have Alzheimer's.

Depression

A study published several years ago in the journal *Neurology* found a strong association between depression and Alzheimer's disease (AD). Researchers collected information on the history of depression among 486 non-demented people ranging in age from 60 to 90, and then followed them for six years, assessing their cognitive function. They found that study participants with a history of depression were 2.5 times more likely to develop AD than people without a history of depression. Previous research has linked depression in older people with early dementia, but it is not yet known whether depression is a cause or a symptom of cognitive problems.

Genetics

Researchers have discovered a number of genes that are associated with heightened risk for AD. The most significant is a variation of a gene called apolipoprotein E (ApoE). ApoE provides instructions for the production of a protein that helps transport cholesterol through the bloodstream and remove it from the body. About 25 percent of the population has at least one copy of ApoE4, a variation of the ApoE gene which has been associated with a higher risk for Alzheimers. Although ApoE4 does not cause Alzheimer's, it may lead to changes in the brain that affect cognitive decline.

"It is not yet clear precisely how ApoE4 affects the brain," says Deborah Blacker, MD. "But it looks like people who have the ApoE4 gene experience a more rapid loss of nerve cell functioning in the frontal lobe, which is important in maintaining higher mental functioning. It might be said that the brains of people with the ApoE4 gene age at a faster rate and that this acceleration may increase the chances of progressing to dementia."

Studies have found that the ApoE4 variation is associated with an increased number of beta-amyloid plaques (protein clumps deposited in the brain), which are a hallmark of Alzheimer's disease. While ApoE may help break down sticky clusters of beta-amyloid protein that can clog the spaces between brain cells, the genetic variation ApoE4 appears to exhibit an impaired ability to degrade beta-amyloid.

"Current research is exploring the gene's role in the creation of plaques and neurofibrillary tangles associated with AD and how it is linked to inflammation, among other things," Dr. Blacker explains.

One particularly innovative study has shed light on how the ApoE-4 variant functions by using a computer model that illustrates its effects. Devised by researchers at the Universitat Autonoma de Barcelona in Spain and the University of Stockholm in Sweden, the model makes it possible to observe the malfunctioning of the APOE-4 variant as it comes into contact with molecules of beta-amyloid. A report on the computer model published in the February 5, 2010 issue of the journal *PLoS Computational Biology,* said the model supports the findings of earlier, more traditional experiments. Because computer modeling is easier to accomplish than conducting in vitro experiments with beta-amyloid, the technique opens up new possibilities for the use of computers in understanding Alzheimer's and other neurological diseases.

There is abundant evidence that people who inherit two copies of ApoE4 have a greater risk of developing Alzheimer's than those who have just one copy. Because not all people with Alzheimer's have this ApoE4 genetic variation, and not all people who have the variation will develop the disease, testing for it currently is not considered a useful predictive tool.

Other genes also appear to play a role in the development of AD. Research suggests that inherited variants of the sortilin-related receptor 1 (SORL1) gene may be involved in the abnormal production of beta-amyloid plaque in the brains of people with late-onset Alzheimer's disease, the most common form of the neurodegenerative disorder. Another genetic factor, a variant of the cell division cycle 2 gene (CDC2), has been associated by Swedish researchers with three times the production of a protein called tau that comprises the neurofibrillary tangles characteristic of Alzheimer's disease. The gene variant was found in half of a group of patients with AD, as opposed to only 35 percent of a group of people without dementia.

At Massachusetts General Hospital, researchers identified four genes that are linked to the development of late-onset Alzheimer's disease. Their work, published in 2008, is the largest genetic analysis of AD carried out to date. A team led by Rudolph Tanzi, PhD, Director of the Genetics and Aging Research Unit at MGH, analyzed genes from hundreds of families with at least three members who had been diagnosed with AD. The investigators screened more than 500,000 gene markers to come up with five genes that seemed closely associated with the onset of AD. Earlier research, as noted above, had already linked one of these genes—the protein APOE4—with increased risk for late-onset AD.

However, four other genes identified by the team were new discoveries. One of these is a DNA marker located on chromosome 14 that is believed to influence the age of disease onset. An analysis comparing 1,400 AD patients with healthy individuals found that the marker was present in many more individuals with AD. A second gene was already known to destroy nerve cells in the central nervous system, leading to a movement disorder called spinocerebellar ataxia. A third gene is thought to be involved in the immune system, and a fourth plays a role in the production of a protein found at the communication points between nerve cells called synapses. The discovery of the new genes is expected to help scientists predict and diagnose AD, and also to deepen understanding of the biochemical events and pathways involved in the disease process.

Since the MGH discoveries, scientific efforts have led to the discovery of a number of other genes associated with increased risk for Alzheimer's disease. These genes—TOMM40, MTHFD1L, and insulin-degrading enzyme (IDE)—are the latest in a growing list of discoveries that may one day lead to diagnosis and treatment of the disease.

A combination of genes and environmental factors may predispose close relatives (brothers, sisters, or children) of Alzheimer's patients to develop the disease as well. The more family members affected by Alzheimer's a person has, the greater the person's risk becomes.

High Blood Pressure

Uncontrolled high blood pressure (hypertension) can lead to stroke—an attack caused by interruption in the blood supply to the brain. Stroke is a major cause of late-life dementia and physical disability. It is the third most common cause of death in the United States, trailing only heart disease and cancer, yet many Americans are unaware that they are at risk, and fail to seek treatment for symptoms that could signal high blood pressure (see Box 4-3) or a brain-damaging cerebral event (see Box 4-4).

Researchers looked for signs of stroke in the brain scans of 2,040 men and women who participated in the long-running Framingham Offspring Study and had undergone magnetic resonance imaging (MRI) scans between 1998 and 2001. They found that, overall, 10.7 percent of participants—whose average age was 62—had suffered silent strokes (transient ischemic attacks, or TIAs). Prevalence among the oldest participants (aged 70 to 89 years) was 15 percent. Although participants were unaware they had suffered a stroke, there was visible evidence of injury to their brains, the researchers said.

"This study emphasizes the risk for silent stroke as we age, and shows how common stroke really is," says staff neurologist Aneesh Singhal, MD, Director of Neurology Quality and Safety at MGH. "It is an excellent reminder that maintaining good brain health as you age requires managing risk factors that can lead to stroke, such as hypertension (high blood pressure), diabetes, high levels of "bad" LDL cholesterol, atrial fibrillation, obesity, and smoking. Knowing the symptoms of stroke and getting immediate medical care for them is also vitally important. "

An interesting new study suggests there may be a relationship between stroke and problems with thinking and memory. The researchers found that older people who do poorly on cognitive tests may be at greater risk for a stroke (see Box 4-5).

Cardiovascular disease

Individuals with cardiovascular disease and heart conditions such as chronic heart failure may have a significantly increased risk of cognitive impairment

Research suggests that the greater the disturbance in blood flow associated with cardiovascular disease (CVD), the greater the decline in cognitive function. A study published a few years ago in the journal *Artery Research*. Correlated measures of performance on neurocognitive tests with ultrasound measurements of blood flow in the circulatory systems of 88 dementia-free older adults with mild to severe CVD. They found a significant association between vascular blood flow levels and neurocognitive function, with poorer blood flow correlated with poorer cognitive functioning, especially in the areas of attention and executive functions such as decision-making and thinking. The authors said their findings suggest that measures of cardiovascular functioning are important markers of risk for common neurocognitive changes, and recommended the development of learning and therapeutic strategies to help individuals with CVD compensate for their neurocognitive limitations.

One type of cardiovascular disease, chronic heart failure (a condition in which the heart is weakened or structurally impaired and cannot meet the body's needs for blood) has been shown to nearly double the incidence of cognitive impairment. However, a program in which people with chronic heart failure were taught strategies to help improve concentration, attention and everyday memory significantly improved cognitive performance in just three months.

Atrial fibrillation, characterized by irregular heart rhythms caused by abnormal electrical impulses in the heart, has also been identified as a significant cause of cognitive decline People with atrial fibrillation (AF) may develop significant cognitive impairment and structural abnormalities of the brain as a result of their condition. Researchers reported in the July 29 issue of the *European Heart Journal* 2009 that a comparison of 122 individuals with AF with a similar group of 563 people without AF revealed significant differences in cognitive performance between the two groups. People with AF scored lower in tasks involving learning, memory, attention, and executive function. Additionally, among people with AF brain scans revealed atrophy of the hippocampus—a region of the brain that plays a key role in memory. Fortunately, effective treatments are available, ranging from simple lifestyle changes (such as reducing consumption of alcohol and caffeine and avoiding medications that contain stimulants) to use of medications or procedures to restore normal heart rhythms or to thin the blood to help prevent clots.

Conditions that damage the heart, such as untreated high blood pressure, diabetes, and high cholesterol, also increase Alzheimer's risk, and many of these risk factors develop early in life. Researchers at Tulane University in New Orleans studied 72 men and women, ages 24 to 44, who were enrolled in the Bogalusa Heart Study. This study has been collecting data on cardiovascular risk factors in African-American and Caucasian children since 1972. The participants were individually given a battery of standard neuropsychological tests that measured verbal ability, reading, number and visual recall, and logical memory. The scores on the tests were then correlated with the participants' cardiovascular risk factors, including blood pressure, age and insulin level.

Results revealed that higher insulin levels negatively impacted logical memory, memory recall and achievement scores, and higher blood pressure scores were associated with poor visual recall scores. The findings emphasize that a healthy brain is dependent upon a healthy heart. The studies in Bogalusa are ongoing, to determine whether this early finding of a link between impaired insulin processing and cognitive dysfunction does, in fact, portend Alzheimer's disease, and whether intervening at an early stage can halt the progression to memory impairment.

Insulin resistance and diabetes

About 40 percent of Americans over age 60 have insulin resistance, a condition in which the cells of the body become less sensitive to the effects of the insulin hormone and have trouble using sugar for energy as a result. This condition is considered a precursor to diabetes. Research finds that high insulin levels may be a major factor in the development of Alzheimer's disease.

Scientists have discovered that the same enzyme that breaks down insulin also breaks down the beta-amyloid protein. When insulin levels are high, the enzyme is occupied with breaking down insulin and can't efficiently clear out beta-amyloid proteins, leading to the deposits in the brain that are a hallmark of Alzheimer's disease. People who have insulin resistance tend to have inflammation and abnormal accumulation of beta-amyloid protein, which are both factors that have been associated with Alzheimer's and other types of dementia.

Some research suggests that people with diabetes are at higher risk for mild cognitive impairment (a possible precursor to Alzheimer's) and are more likely to develop dementia and Alzheimer's disease, even after controlling for other vascular problems—especially if they are older. The cognitive effects of the disease appear early and continue into old age, recent research suggests. Individuals with diabetes do not perform as well as healthy people in tests of several key brain functions, according to a report in the January 2009 issue of the journal *Neuropsychology*. Researchers compared the results of cognitive tests taken by adults between the ages of 53 and 90 who participated in a large longitudinal study. Forty-one of the participants had diabetes and 424 were healthy. The investigators found that while both groups of participants performed similarly on tests of episodic memory (recollections of events, times and places related to a person's history) and semantic memory (memory for words and their meanings and generic information), there were significant differences between the two groups in tests of executive function, and in speed of information processing. The differences were found to appear early in the course of diabetes and remain stable. The study authors suggest that people with diabetes should manage the disorder with diet and medications and have their cognitive abilities monitored.

If people with diabetes fail to control their blood sugar, they may face an even greater risk of dementia. Researchers at Kaiser Permanente in northern California studied nearly 23,000 people over the age of 50 with type 2 diabetes to determine the link between glycosylated hemoglobin readings (a blood test that assesses blood sugar levels over time) and dementia. A normal reading is seven or below. Results suggested that the higher the patients' glycosylated hemoglobin, the greater their dementia risk. The study did not find any correlation between dementia and diabetes when levels remained below 10, but readings above that level began to impact dementia risk. Participants whose glycosylated hemoglobin results were between 12 and 14.9 had a 24 percent higher dementia risk, and those with a reading over 15 had an 83 percent higher risk for dementia than those with normal readings.

Severe low levels of blood sugar (hypoglycemia) are also damaging to the brain. In a study of 16,667 older patients with type 2 diabetes, researchers found that people who experienced one episode of low blood sugar that required hospitalization were 26 percent more likely to develop dementia than people with diabetes who had never experienced an episode. Increased risk rose to 80 percent among people who experienced two episodes, and to 94 percent in people who had three episodes or more.

There is some evidence that taking chromium picolinate, a supplement that combines chromium with picolinic acid, might provide some benefit for elderly adults with signs of memory decline (see Box 4-6). The supplement is thought to improve glucose metabolism in the brain, resulting in improved brain function.

Head injury

Although not everyone who experiences head trauma goes on to develop Alzheimer's, research is finding that head injury can increase Alzheimer's risk. A brain injury leads to the formation of beta-amyloid deposits in the brain, which can accelerate the development of Alzheimer's. Traumatic brain injury can lead to permanent cognitive impairment related to the area of damage.

Lack of education

A lack of education may interfere with more than job prospects. Research has indicated that a more robust education may help people build up a "cognitive reserve" that enables them to deal with the debilitating cognitive effects of Alzheimer's. In one 2003 study, Alzheimer's patients with more formal education scored higher on tests of cognitive abilities, irrespective of how much beta-amyloid plaque was in their brains. More recent research may help explain why: Higher levels of education are associated with larger brains, and larger brains appear to be more resistant to the debilitating effects of AD.

Several studies have linked a bigger brain to lower risk for Alzheimer's disease (AD), even in individuals with large amounts of the plaques and tangles characteristic of the neurological disorder. In one investigation, scientists conducted postmortem examinations of the brains of 36 older adults, 24 of whom had symptoms of AD, when they died, and 12 of whom were dementia-free. The researchers found that all of the brains they examined had large amounts of beta-amyloid plaque and neurofibrillary tangles normally associated with AD and were similar in most other respects. But there was a significant difference between the two groups in a key memory region of the brain. This region, called the hippocampus, was on average 20 percent bigger in the 12 people who had stayed mentally sharp all their lives than it was in the people who developed dementia. The findings suggest that a larger hippocampus may protect people from the effects of Alzheimer's disease-related brain changes that often accompany aging, such as beta-amyloid plaque and neurofibrillary tangles, and may point the way to new prevention strategies.

Other research suggests that while having a greater cognitive reserve may not prevent the development of plaques and tangles associated with AD, it may help people cope better with their memory disorder. Researchers injected a radio-carbon-labeled compound formulated to attach itself to clusters of beta-amyloid plaque into the brains of 37 people with AD and 161 people without dementia. They then used positron emission tomography (PET) technology to perform scans of the determine the size of the plaque clusters in each participant's brain. Study participants also took tests to assess cognitive performance. Results showed an association between education and cognitive performance among people with high levels of plaques in the brain: The more education these individuals had, the fewer their symptoms of dementia. Education played no role in cognitive performance among people with low levels of plaque. The findings suggest that a higher educational level may help individuals cope with Alzheimer's pathology and delay symptoms of dementia. The results do not indicate whether people can do anything to boost cognitive reserve later in life the authors said, but suggested that "it doesn't hurt to remain active, physically as well as mentally."

Poor diet

A diet high in fat and low in important nutrients can lead to a cascade of events that ultimately contribute to Alzheimer's. Unhealthy diets can lead to chemical changes in the brain, accumulation of excess abdominal fat, high blood pressure, and high insulin levels, among other effects. These risk factors may, in turn, contribute to health conditions such as diabetes and stroke, which have been directly associated with increased Alzheimer's risk.

Animal studies suggest that eating foods loaded with fat, sugar and cholesterol may increase your risk of developing Alzheimer's disease. Mice engineered to be susceptible to AD were fed a junk food diet for nine months, after which their brains were examined. Researchers found that the mouse brains exhibited chemical changes similar to changes that occur in the Alzheimer brain, suggesting that a high intake of fat and cholesterol in combination with genetic factors may adversely affect brain chemicals and contribute to the development of AD. The changes included an abnormal build-up of the protein tau that is found in neurofibrillary tangles associated with the memory disorder, as well as depletion of a protein called Arc that is necessary to memory storage.

Box 4-7: Memory decline gets worse with stress

Stress can speed up memory decline in people whose cognitive functioning is already impaired. That's the conclusion of a recent study that followed 52 adults ages 65 to 97 over a three-year period. Researchers compared 27 individuals whose cognitive functioning was impaired at the outset of the study to 25 individuals who had no cognitive impairment when the study began. The 27 individuals who showed signs of cognitive impairment at the outset of the study had a higher incidence of memory deterioration during they study if they reported experiencing a stressful life event (such as the death of a loved one or hospitalization) in the past six to 12 months. In contrast, the 25 people who were unimpaired at the outset of the study showed no memory decline, even when they reported exposure to similar stressors, according to a report in the December 2009 *American Journal of Psychiatry*.

Smoking

Studies indicate that smoking can dramatically increase a person's risk of developing dementia. In one investigation, researchers followed almost 7,000 people age 55 and older for an average of seven years. During that time, 706 participants developed dementia. People who smoked were 50 percent more likely to develop Alzheimer's disease or other forms of dementia than those who didn't smoke or who had smoked in the past but had quit.

Even inhaling second-hand smoke can affect cognition. An analysis of data on more than 4,800 nonsmokers over the age of 50 suggests that people exposed to secondhand smoke may face a 44 percent increased risk of developing dementia. In the largest study to date showing an association between exposure to tobacco smoke and the development of dementia, researchers tested saliva samples for levels of cotinine, a by-product of nicotine, and evaluated participants' performance on tests of verbal, math and memory skills. They found that the higher the levels of cotinine a participant had the greater his or her risk for cognitive impairment: those with the highest cotinine levels had a 44 percent increased risk of cognitive impairment compared with those with the lowest cotinine levels. In a report in the February 13, 2009 online edition of the journal *BMJ*, study authors said the findings indicate that passive smoking may be nearly as bad for health as active smoking and suggested that nonsmokers stay away from areas where people smoke.

Smoking is thought to affect memory by increasing the risk of cardiovascular disease (a known risk factor for dementia), or by damaging blood vessels and increasing the likelihood of hardening of the arteries. The tobacco habit also can damage brain cells and stop new cells from forming. Studies show that smokers do not remember names and faces as well as non-smokers.

Stress

Too much stress can make mild memory problems worse, according to a recent study, possibly because of damage to brain cells caused by high levels of stress hormones (See Box 4-7). ◼

5 DETECTING ALZHEIMER'S

Considering that finding Alzheimer's early can help you get treatment and possibly slow the progression of the disease, one of the most crucial areas of Alzheimer's research today is finding new ways to diagnose the disease while it's still in its early stages. Although no definitive test for Alzheimer's exists, researchers are making great strides in understanding how the disease begins and progresses.

"We are definitely making progress in diagnosing Alzheimer's disease," says Bruce H. Price, MD, Chief of the Department of Neurology at McLean Hospital in Boston, and an associate neurologist at Massachusetts General Hospital. "People who are worried about memory problems or loss of concentration should be seen as soon as possible by a neurologist, geriatric psychiatrist or other expert who specializes in the diagnosis of AD. Early detection allows patients and their families to plan for treatment and care, and make informed decisions together about the future."

Knowing the warning signs

Watch out for these 10 warning signs from the Alzheimer's Association's checklist of common symptoms. Contact your doctor right away if you experience:
- Recent memory loss that affects job skills
- Difficulty performing familiar tasks
- Problems with language
- Disorientation of time and place
- Poor or decreased judgment
- Problems with abstract thinking
- Misplacing things
- Changes in mood or behavior
- Changes in personality
- Loss of initiative

Diagnosing Alzheimer's

Because there is not one specialist for Alzheimer's, getting a diagnosis begins with a visit to your general practitioner. You also may be seen by a neurologist, psychiatrist or psychologist.

Your doctor will review your medical history, ask you about any symptoms you've experienced, review any medications you might be taking, and give you

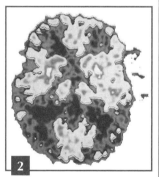
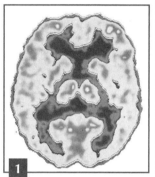
a physical exam. You also may be asked to take a battery of neuropsychological tests to measure aspects of brain function such as memory, attention, executive functions (such as problem-solving abilities, calculation and abstraction) language skills, and visuo-spacial abilities.

Doctors generally arrive at an Alzheimer's diagnosis by eliminating other possible causes of dementia. Even if another cause for the dementia is not found, diagnosing and managing conditions such as infection, high blood pressure, cardiovascular disease, depression, and other problems that can compromise brain function is an important aspect of dementia treatment. Your doctor may give you one or more of the following diagnostic and cognitive function tests:

- **Mini mental state examination (MMSE).** Your doctor will ask you a series of questions, such as the names of common objects, the date, the location of your doctor's office, or to follow an instruction. The maximum score on the MMSE is 30 points. A score of 20 to 24 suggests mild dementia, 13 to 19 suggests moderate dementia, and 12 or less indicates severe dementia.

- **Montreal cognitive assessment test (MoCA).** MoCA is a more sensitive test than the MMSE especially for MCI and mild or early onset AD. Like the MMSE, it involves 30 points and takes only 10 minutes to complete but is available in more than 10 languages. MoCA has 100 percent sensitivity in detecting mild AD and 90 percent sensitivity in detecting MCI.

- **Mini-cog.** This test asks you to remember three common objects and then repeat them a few minutes later, as well as to draw a clock showing a time your doctor specifies.

- **Blood and urine tests.** These tests can rule out medical conditions that cause memory loss, such as thyroid problems, kidney or liver dysfunction, or infection.

- **Neurological test.** Your doctor will check your coordination, balance, eye movement, speech and reflexes.

- **Brain imaging.** Your doctor may recommend one or more of the available brain imaging techniques to help arrive at a diagnosis. Computed tomography (CT) provides a three-dimensional view of your brain to help your doctor identify a stroke or intracranial hemorrhage. Magnetic resonance imaging (MRI) identifies abnormalities in brain structure with sharper resolution than CT scans, and can help doctors assess the structure of your brain. Positron emission tomography (PET) and a new application for MRI called functional MRI (fMRI) can assess how well the cells of your brain are functioning (see Box 5-1).

New tests for Alzheimer's

A careful clinical diagnosis is more than 90 percent accurate in diagnosing Alzheimer's disease. But researchers are working to identify new ways to detect Alzheimer's in its initial stages and help accurately distinguish between Alzheimer's disease and other forms of dementia. Earlier diagnosis will help ensure that as new and better treatments become available, patients may be able to benefit from them before the brain has been irreparably damaged.

A major initiative aimed at identifying AD in its earliest stages promises to help in the quest for new drugs that can slow or stop the disease before major damage has been done to the brain. The initiative, a large study supported by the U.S. National Institute on Aging and other public and private entities, is called the Alzheimer's Disease Neuroimaging Initiative (ADNI). Begun in 2004, the ongoing $60 million study tracks more than 800 individuals with AD and mild cognitive impairment (MCI is often a precursor to AD). Participants are assessed for a number of biomarkers, such as changes in brain structure and body chemistry that can be used in combination with clinical and neuropsychological measures to track the progress of AD. A number of scientists have built on ADNI data to find diagnostic approaches that detect AD with a high degree of reliability.

"The studies coming out of the ADNI initiative are among the most clinically important research initiatives we have seen," says neuropsychiatrist Kaloyan Tanev, MD, of the Neuropsychiatry Clinic at Massachusetts General Hospital. "The researchers are testing tools that could be used in clinical settings. These are effective methods for identifying AD that may well be available for use in ordinary medical practice within a matter of years. It's very exciting."

Here are a few promising tests for Alzheimer's currently in the pipeline:

Brain scans

Neuroimaging can help assess activity in various brain regions, and new research suggests that neuroimaging techniques such as magnetic resonance imaging (MRI) and positron emission tomography (PET) can detect signs of changes in the brain structure of living people that may be associated with early Alzheimer's disease. Brain scanning techniques currently being investigated focus primarily on two procedures: brain scans to test the volume of key brain regions, and brain scans to detect glucose activity levels in key brain regions. The findings might one day lead to new diagnostic tests for AD.

Researchers at New York University School of Medicine and Ambient, Inc. used PET scans to identify areas of the brain in which glucose metabolism had declined. Although earlier studies have found that impaired glucose metabolism,

Box 5-2: Scans find differences in glucose metabolism in early- vs. late-onset AD

Researchers set out to determine why early age-of-onset Alzheimer's disease (AD) is associated with more rapid disease progression, more generalized cognitive deficits, greater brain atrophy and slower metabolism compared to late-onset AD at a similar disease stage. The investigators used sophisticated brain imaging techniques to detect a key difference between biological mechanisms involved in early-onset Alzheimer's disease (AD)—which is associated with the presence of the APoE-4 gene variation—and late-onset AD. The scientists divided 39 individuals with AD according to age at first symptoms into two groups, those who were younger than 65 years of age, and those who were older. A third group of healthy individuals were recruited as a control group. Investigators examined the brains of all participants using positron emission tomography (PET) scans with Pittsburgh compound-B, a marker that binds with toxic beta-amyloid plaque in the brain, and a second mildly radioactive substance that marked the presence of glucose in brain cells. PET scans of the three participant groups revealed that compared to normal participants, both AD groups had increased burdens of beta-amyloid plaque in the frontal, parietal and lateral temporal cortices of their brains at similar stages in the disease process, with no significant differences between the two groups in plaque load. However, compared with participants with late-onset AD, the early-onset individuals revealed significantly lower glucose metabolism (indicating a decline in activity) in the posterior cortical region, which is involved in sensory awareness. The results suggest that the more rapid progression of disease in early-onset AD may be linked to early beta-amyloid accumulation and increased vulnerability to beta-amyloid pathology as indicated by slower glucose metabolism in key brain areas.

particularly in the hippocampus, may be a significant marker for AD, this important memory region is difficult to measure with conventional analysis techniques. The researchers developed an automated method using PET scans to rapidly and accurately sample glucose metabolism in many areas of the brain including the hippocampus. They used this technique to determine which of 32 brain regions was most predictive of disease progression as confirmed by subsequent tests of memory and thinking. They found that employing the automated technique to identify low levels of glucose metabolism in the hippocampus might be a sensitive predictor of disease progression, and might be useful for diagnosis of AD. Compared to healthy individuals, people with stable MCI had a 12 percent reduction in glucose metabolism, people with MCI with subsequent clinical decline had a 14 percent reduction, and people with AD had a 24 percent reduction in glucose metabolism.

"Predicting subsequent cognitive decline by looking for low levels of glucose metabolism in key brain regions with automated PET scans could be useful to clinicians, and could be made widely available to them in a relatively short time frame," comments Dr. Tanev.

A recently developed technique using PET scans to detect the accumulation of beta-amyloid plaque—a marker for Alzheimer's disease—in the brains of living people is already being used to help scientists increase their understanding of the disease (see Box 5-2). The procedure involves injecting individuals with an innovative fluorescent tracer called Pittsburgh Compound-B (PiB). The tracer crosses the blood/brain barrier to bind with beta-amyloid plaque in the brain, making it visible in the scans. The technique holds promise for research and for use in diagnosing and treating patients. Massachusetts General Hospital has been involved in the development of the imaging agent used for those purposes.

In a study of another scanning technique, researchers used a specially designed semi-automated magnetic resonance imaging technique to identify individuals with mild cognitive impairment (MCI) who are most likely to progress to Alzheimer's disease (AD). The imaging made it possible to discern subtle anatomic alterations in the brain that signal atrophy. The investigators used the imaging to analyze images from 175 people with MCI, 84 people with mild Alzheimer's disease, and 139 healthy controls. In follow-up with 160 of the subjects with MCI, the researchers found that individuals whose brain atrophy patterns most resembled the atrophy patterns of the subjects with mild AD were more likely to experience significant one-year clinical declines and structural brain loss, and were more likely to progress to a probable diagnosis of AD than individuals who did not show these patterns. The atrophy patterns affected regions of the medial and lateral temporal lobes of the brain (responsible for comprehension and verbal memory, among other functions), and the frontal lobes (responsible for functions such as reasoning and planning), according to a report in February 2009 in the online edition of the journal *Radiology*.

Scientists from Trinity College in Dublin, Ireland, have found that magnetic resonance imaging (MRI) volume measurements of the left hippocampus—a section of the brain associated with memory and AD—used in combination with three specific memory tests could predict with 94 percent accuracy which individuals with MCI would go on to develop Alzheimer's disease.

In another study, researchers at the University of California, San Diego School of Medicine developed a fully computerized neuroimaging technique to assess how changes in brain volume correlated with worsening cognitive status. The automated system, called Volumetric MRI, rapidly measures brain changes in memory centers of the brain such as the hippocampus, amygdala and temporal horn and compares them with the size of these regions in healthy individuals. Individuals with smaller measurements in the hippocampus and amygdala, and larger measurements in the temporal horn were found to decline more rapidly on tests assessing cognitive decline and dementia, suggesting that structural brain changes in these regions might be a reliable predictor of progression to AD.

"These methods appear to be highly predictive, but they are not yet clinically available," says Dr. Tanev. "However, software that simplifies the use of MRI for measuring brain volume and that is fast, accurate and easy to use will increase the likelihood that these techniques may be available to clinicians and their patients in a matter of a few years."

Biomarkers

Studies have identified a pattern of 23 protein biomarkers found in cerebrospinal fluid (the fluid surrounding the brain and spinal cord) that may help devise a new test for Alzheimer's. In research, this pattern was found in 93 percent of Alzheimer's patients, although some individuals without Alzheimer's also exhibited the pattern.

Other research involving biomarkers suggests that an abnormal combination of two proteins in the spinal fluid of people with cognitive impairment may also lead to a diagnostic test for AD. Researchers measured levels of the proteins—an enzyme call prostaglandin-d-synthase and a protein called transthyretin—in post-mortem examinations of four people with mild cognitive impairment and eight people who had late-stage Alzheimer's diseases. They then compared the results with post-mortem levels of the combination in people who had no signs of cognitive impairment. The investigation revealed much higher levels of the protein complex in people with cognitive impairment. In subsequent measurements of the cerebrospinal fluid of 15 living people with probable AD and 14 healthy individuals the researchers found that probable AD participants had six times the levels of the protein complex as the healthy subjects. In a report in the June 6, 2008 online edition of the journal *Neurology*, the study authors suggested that measuring levels of the protein combination "may allow identification of subjects with Alzheimer's disease early in the disease."

Still another effort to find biomarkers that signal the early stages of Alzheimer's disease involves assessing cerebrospinal fluid (CSF) for the protein beta-amyloid 42 (which forms the plaque associated with AD), and a type of tau identified as P-tau (a source of the neurofibrillary tangles associated with AD). Researchers found that low levels of beta-amyloid 42 and high levels of P-tau were correlated with early AD in many individuals. The CSF assessment predicted AD in 62 percent of individuals, and accurately ruled out AD in 88 percent of cases. Another, smaller, study, found among 49 older patients with MCI, those who had lower levels of beta-amyloid 42 and higher levels of tau and P-tau were more likely to progress rapidly to AD.

"Studies of biomarkers are interesting from a research standpoint because they may tell us more about the mechanisms that are involved in the disease process," says Dr. Tanev. "However they involve invasive procedures to obtain spinal fluid and may not be as accurate in identifying people in the early stages of the disease as the brain scans mentioned earlier."

Smell test

Researchers have found that difficulty identifying several common scents, among them lemon and banana, may herald the onset of Alzheimer's. People in one study who scored lower on a 12-item smell-identification test tended to have increased numbers of Alzheimer's-associated tangles in their brain. Recently, scientists discovered the underlying processes that lead to these changes in mice bred to develop AD (see Box 5-3). Eventually, a "scratch-and-sniff" test might help doctors identify people with Alzheimer's. Other research may lead to the development of an eye test that signals the early stages of AD (see Box 5-4).

Blood test

Certain proteins may be present at higher levels in the blood of people with Alzheimer's. Finding methods to detect these proteins may one day lead to an effective diagnostic test for AD. One method developed several years ago uses molecular tests to detect changes in 18 of more than 120 proteins used by cells to communicate with one another. The changes appear to be related to changes in the brain accompanying Alzheimer's disease—a finding that might provide the basis for an accurate diagnostic test. The molecular tests have been successful in detecting AD with 91 percent accuracy as many as two to six years before obvious symptoms appear. This promising finding may one day lead to the development of a blood test to help identify Alzheimer's, monitor the course of treatment, and contribute to the development of new medications.

Alzheimer's prediction method

Researchers at the Karolinska Institute in Stockholm, Sweden, have developed an Alzheimer's prediction method based on data from the Cardiovascular Risk Factors, Aging and Dementia study, which included 1,409 middle-aged Finnish people. To determine Alzheimer's risk, the researchers assign a score to each of the following risk factors: age, education, gender, systolic blood pressure, body mass index, blood cholesterol and physical activity. By combining the scores, the researchers say they can identify people at high risk for developing dementia within the following 20 years, so that those people can implement lifestyle changes early. Researchers are continuing to fine-tune the test, and to determine whether altering these risk factors will actually change dementia outcomes.

Researchers at the University of California in San Francisco have formulated a new tool that estimates an older adult's risk of AD. The list includes many well-known risk factors for the disease, including genetic susceptibility, poor performance on tests of thinking skills, and older age, but also includes factors such as having had a coronary bypass surgery, being slow at physical tasks, and being underweight. A score of 8 or more on the 15-point scale indicates increased risk for dementia. In a six-year study of more than 3,000 participants with an average age of 76, the prediction tool correctly classified 88 percent of the participants with respect to dementia risk, according to a report on the study published online on May 13, 2009 in the journal *Neurology*. The results showed that 56 per cent of participants with high scores on the risk index developed dementia, compared with 23 per cent who only had moderate scores and 4 per cent who had low scores. ■

NEW FINDING

Box 5-4: Finding may lead to eye test for Alzheimer's disease

Researchers say their work suggests that an amyloid protein that accumulates in the lens of the eyes of people with Down syndrome may also signal the presence of early Alzheimer's disease (AD). In a study published In the May 20, 2010 issue of the journal *PLoS One*, the scientists found that the protein triggers an accumulation of toxic beta-amyloid, a hallmark of Alzheimer's disease, and causes the characteristic supranuclear cataracts that appear only in people with advanced AD and Down syndrome. The researchers are currently developing an eye scanner they hope will measure beta-amyloid in the lens of the eye as a way to provide early detection and monitoring of related pathology in the brain.

6 TREATING ALZHEIMER'S

There is no question that over the long term, Alzheimer's can have a devastating effect on a person's quality of life. Although no cure exists for the disease, treatments can improve some of the most troublesome cognitive and behavioral symptoms, and perhaps slow progression of the disease. New treatments on the horizon may offer even greater relief—and one day possibly a cure—for Alzheimer's.

Alzheimer's medications

Drugs used to treat Alzheimer's can be divided into two categories. One category treats memory, language skills, and other cognitive symptoms of the disease, while the other addresses agitation and other behavioral issues. Cholinesterase inhibitors and memantine (Namenda) both treat cognitive symptoms.

Cholinesterase inhibitors

These drugs boost levels of a brain chemical called acetylcholine, a neurotransmitter essential for proper memory function that is reduced in people with Alzheimer's. All of the drugs in this class appear to be about equally effective. Most cholinesterase inhibitors can slow the progression of mild-to-moderate Alzheimer's in about half of the people who take them. One, Aricept, is also approved for use with severe AD. Side effects of these drugs are generally mild, and include nausea, vomiting and upset stomach.

Cholinesterase inhibitors commonly used for people with Alzheimer's include:

- Donepezil (Aricept): Taken once a day and is indicated for use with mild to severe Alzheimer's. Research has shown that the medication helped memory in patients with moderate-to-severe Alzheimer's.
- Rivastigmine (Exelon): Taken twice daily with food in oral form. A once-a-day skin patch version of Exelon recently received approval by the U.S. Food and Drug Administration (FDA). The patch is associated with fewer side effects than oral Exelon and is helpful in treating patients who have trouble swallowing. The patch also has been approved to treat dementia related to Parkinson's disease.
- Galantamine (Razadyne): This drug has been shown to improve mental function and behavior in patients with mild-to-moderate Alzheimer's, as well as in those who have both Alzheimer's and vascular dementia. An extended-release version can be given just once a day.

- N-methyl-D-aspartate (NMDA) glutamate receptor antagonist: This drug is neuroprotective and reduces the excititoxity of the cell due to excessive exposure or over stimulation of NMDA that may led to cell death. However normal NMDA activity is necessary for cellular function and blocking all activity would cause unacceptable side effects. Only one such drug is available and approved for use in Alzheimer's at this time.

- Memantine (Namenda): Approved in 2003 to treat moderate-to-severe Alzheimer's, this drug blocks the action of a chemical messenger in the brain called glutamate, which in excess can damage nerve cells. When used alone or together with Aricept and possibly other cholinesterase inhibitors, Namenda can delay Alzheimer's progression and improve cognitive function in some patients. The most common side effects are constipation, drowsiness, dizziness, and headache.

Combination therapy

Scientists at Massachusetts General Hospital (MGH) have provided concrete evidence that long-term therapy pairing the drug memantine (Namenda, Ebixa) with cholinesterase inhibitors—including galantamine (Reminyl), donepezil (Aricept) and rivastigmine (Exelon)—appears to be more beneficial with time and works substantially better than either class of drug used alone. MGH researchers studied the long-term effects of combined treatment with memantine (Namenda) and cholinesterase inhibitor medication (such as galantamine [Reminy] donepezil [Aricept] and rivastigmine [Exelon]) either alone or in combination, and followed a variety of patients in all stages of the disease. Using clinical data on 382 people with AD, the scientists analyzed treatment modalities, memory performance and measures of daily functioning among study participants over the years 1990 to 2005. Of the group, 144 people received no drug treatment for their AD, 122 received treatment with cholinesterase inhibitors alone, and 116 received treatment with both memantine and cholinesterase inhibitors. Researchers found that all of the AD patients declined over the course of the study, but that those treated with a combination of memantine and cholinesterase inhibitors did better, experiencing benefits in measures of cognition and daily living. The rate of decline among patients who received combination treatment was slower and the longer they received treatment, the greater the effect. The beneficial effects of the treatment affected patients at all stages and persisted for years, the study authors reported.

Results of their multi-year study suggest the drug combination is the most effective treatment to date for the progressive disorder—and the findings are expected to change the way patients with AD are treated.

"We don't yet have a cure for Alzheimer's disease, but now it's no longer accurate to say we don't have a useful treatment," says Alireza Atri, MD, PhD, of the MGH Department of Neurology, lead author of the study. "Our research found real benefits that last a number of years in real-life settings with real patients. The results suggest that if you want to give yourself or a loved one the best chance of slowing symptoms of the disease, long-term combination therapy is the best currently available option. While for most people treatment expectations are modest, they do translate, in the long-term, to clinically significant benefits that are likely to positively affect quality of life for patients and their families and caregivers."

Behavioral and psychiatric symptoms can be especially troublesome for people with Alzheimer's disease and their caretakers. Symptoms such as anxiety, agitation, hallucinations, delusions, aggression, hostility and uncooperativeness are among the most important reasons that people with Alzheimer's are institutionalized.

Non-drug approaches may be effective in easing behavioral problems—for example, discovering and addressing the causes of distress, assessing the person's drug regimen to see if current medications may be affecting behavior, distracting the person, creating a peaceful environment, and simplifying tasks. If these approaches are not successful, medications may help. Although no drugs have been approved by the FDA specifically to treat behavioral and psychiatric symptoms of Alzheimer's, several have shown some efficacy when used off-label. These medications include:

Antidepressants

Antidepressants known as selective serotonin reuptake inhibitors (SSRIs) can help slow cognitive decline in people with Alzheimer's who have symptoms of depression, research shows. SSRIs such as fluoxetine (Prozac), paroxetine (Paxil), sertraline (Zoloft), and others can ease irritability and depression in people with Alzheimer's. Research suggests older adults with AD with symptoms of depression who are continuously treated with antidepressants may have less cognitive decline than those whose depression is not treated or only treated intermittently.

Antipsychotic medications

Inappropriate verbal, vocal or motor activity affects up to 70 percent of individuals with dementia. This agitated behavior may take a number of forms, including irritability, pacing, searching, repetitive speech, insatiable demands for attention, anger, shouting, or hitting. "Off label" treatment with antipsychotic medications was a common therapeutic response to these behaviors until recent studies called this treatment into question, especially for periods longer than 12 weeks or so. In a study published in the January 8, 2009 online issue of

The Lancet Neurology, researchers reported that prolonged use of antipsychotics in older patients nearly doubles the risk of patient death over three years. The researchers followed 165 Alzheimer's patients ages 67 to 100 who were treated with either antipsychotic drugs or placebo. Over time, health outcomes for the two groups showed increasing differences, with 72 percent of patients taking placebo surviving at 24 months versus 46 percent of patients taking antipsychotics, and 59 percent of patients taking placebo surviving at 36 months versus 30 percent of patients taking antipsychotic drugs.

"In light of these findings, antipsychotic treatment of dementia-related agitation has been reevaluated," says Maurizio Fava, MD, Vice Chair of the Department of Psychiatry at MGH. "Antipsychotic drugs such as haloperidol (Haldol), olanzapine (Zyprexa) risperidone (Risperdal) and quetiapine (Seroquel) still may be used for short periods of time without undue risk in cases of extreme agitation or aggression when other measures do not work. But use for longer periods is not recommended in most patients."

Instead of turning to antipsychotic medications at the first sign of agitation, Dr. Fava recommends approaching behavioral issues on a on a case-by-case basis, using a range of possible strategies that reflect the specific circumstances and characteristics of the person with dementia. There are a number of possible non-pharmacological options for calming an agitated person, including:

- **Avoiding potentially upsetting situations:** It may be possible to forestall agitation by anticipating and resolving factors—such as boredom, excessive stimulation or pain—that seem to cause disruptive behaviors.

- **Allowing for some agitation:** Certain behaviors might be allowed rather than restricted, provided they do not complicate caregiving or pose a risk to the person with dementia or others. For example, a person with dementia for whom a sense of independence is important might be encouraged to perform basic functions such as selecting a wardrobe, even when this results in odd clothing combinations.

- **Responding flexibly:** Allow for changes in routine and environment to help keep the older person calm. For example, a type of food that is often rejected by the person with dementia could be replaced with an equally nourishing food that is more acceptable to the individual.

"You can also seek advice from support groups to help you find safe ways to cope with disturbed behavior," Dr. Fava advises. "But if these basic measures do not work to control agitation, don't hesitate to seek professional help. A health care provider may recommend alternatives to riskier antipsychotic drugs that have been shown to help soothe some agitated individuals, such as cholinesterase inhibitors used to treat dementia, antidepressants such as trazodone (Desyrel) and selective serotonin reuptake inhibitors (SSRIs), anti-epileptic medications such as divalproex (Depakote), and lithium. If your loved one is being treated with antipsychotics, share your concerns about the medication with his or her care provider."

In circumstances in which people with Alzheimer's develop severe behavioral problems such as hallucinations, delusions or aggression that do not respond to other therapies, it may be necessary to prescribe antipsychotic drugs in the short term until other, less risky, strategies can be found. Because the older antipsychotic medications such as haloperidol (Haldol) can have significant side effects—such as muscle spasms, insomnia, and agitation—doctors tend to prescribe a newer class of drugs known as atypical antipsychotic medications, which include risperidone (Risperdal), olanzapine (Zyprexa), and others.

"Despite serious concerns, a case still can be made for the use of antipsychotic medications under certain circumstances," says Dr. Fava. "In certain patients, the medications can help reduce some of the worst behavioral symptoms of AD. This is important because unmanageable behavior often triggers a move from home care to a nursing home, where antipsychotics may be necessary to prevent an unstable patient from harming another resident."

Other drugs

Doctors also use anxiolytics, or anti-anxiety drugs, such as lorazepam (Ativan) and oxazepam (Serax) to reduce the anxiety and disruptive symptoms of Alzheimer's. Some research has shown that medications used in epilepsy treatment such as carbamazepine (Tegretol) and divalproex sodium (Depakote) may successfully reduce agitation and aggression in some Alzheimer's patients, although other research does not support this finding.

Alternative treatments

Several alternative treatments have been investigated for the prevention, slowing, or treatment of Alzheimer's and dementia. However, it's important to be cautious and consult your doctor before using any type of supplement, because they are not regulated by the FDA, and even so-called "natural" supplements can sometimes cause side effects. Moreover, the potency and purity of supplements are not guaranteed.

Coenzyme Q10

Coenzyme Q10 (CoQ10) is an antioxidant compound that is made naturally by the body and is found in most foods. It is essential to cellular energy production and to the control of cell-damaging free radicals that are created as a by-product of that production. Preliminary evidence suggests that this supplement may slow Alzheimer's-related dementia, but this has yet to be confirmed. What's more, the supplement is very expensive—about $100 a month for a low dose of 300 mg a day—and strength and quality can vary significantly among various brands.

A number of side effects have been associated with CoQ10, although most are mild and of short duration. They include headache, dizziness, insomnia, nausea, gastrointestinal upset, rash, fatigue, irritability, and lowered blood pressure and blood sugar levels. People with diabetes or hypoglycemia and those taking blood pressure medication should check with their health-care providers before taking the supplement.

Ginkgo biloba

Ginkgo biloba is believed to have both antioxidant and anti-inflammatory properties, and the supplement is commonly used as an Alzheimer's treatment in Europe. Some research has shown modest cognitive improvements in patients with early-stage Alzheimer's disease (AD) who took the herbal supplement, but the largest study to date suggests that the supplements may provide no benefit at all.

The long-lasting study of the effects of ginkgo biloba on dementia risk concluded that the ginkgo biloba neither wards off nor slows the progression of Alzheimer's disease (AD) and other age-related dementias. Researchers recruited more than 3,000 adults 75 and older who showed no signs of AD at the outset of the investigation, and treated half of the group with daily doses of ginkgo biloba and half with an inactive placebo. Over a period of about six years, 523 participants were diagnosed with dementia, 277 (18 percent) in the ginkgo group, and 246 (16 percent) in the placebo group, according to information published in the November 19, 2008 and December 30, 2009 issues of the *Journal of the American Medical Association*. The differences between the two groups were not considered significant. The researchers found no effect on the progression of mild cognitive impairment (MCI) to dementia, suggesting the supplement does not slow development of disease. There was no difference between people who took the herb and those who took placebo in any cognitive domains, including memory, attention, visuospatial abilities, language, and executive functions (decision-making and planning). Investigators did find a slight increase in risk of hemorrhagic (bleeding) strokes among people who took ginkgo biloba, especially in combination with blood-thinning drugs such as aspirin and warfarin (Coumadin). But again, the small difference was not considered significant.

"Based on this research, ginkgo biloba cannot be recommended for preventing dementia," the lead researcher concluded.

Huperzine A

Huperzine A is a natural version of the cholinesterase inhibitors derived from the moss Huperzia serrata. It has been used for centuries in Chinese traditional medicine. Studies suggest that its effects may be similar to that of the cholinesterase inhibitors, and it should not be used together with these drugs. Huperzine A is generally safe and well-tolerated, although it may increase the risk of having seizures for individuals with epilepsy and has caused changes in heart rhythm in some individuals. Other, milder, side effects include stomach cramps, nausea and diarrhea, sweating, blurry vision and dizziness. The supplement is still being studied to see if it has benefit for Alzheimer's.

Omega-3 fatty acids

Omega-3 fatty acids—found in algae and fatty cold-water fish such as salmon, mackerel, sardines, trout, and tuna—have been linked to a reduced risk of heart disease and stroke, and some evidence suggests that they also may help prevent dementia. A number of theories have been advanced to explain the possible protective effect of omega-3s on memory. It Is thought that omega-3 fatty acids have beneficial effects on blood vessels and inflammation, and may possibly stimulate the growth of dendrites, branches that protrude from neurons and connect nerve cells to one another. A large study of 3,660 people 65 and older suggests that consuming plenty of fish rich in omega-3 fatty acids may help protect the brain against strokes and silent brain infarcts (multiple small strokes) that have been linked to cognitive decline and dementia. Researchers questioned participants about the fish in their diets, and used imaging technology to scan their brains for signs of brain lesions. The brain scans were repeated five years later on 2,313 of the participants, at which point consumption of fish was correlated with the number of brain lesions each participant had. The investigation showed that compared to individuals who did not eat fish regularly, individuals who ate broiled or baked fish high in omega-3 fatty acids at least three times a week were 26 percent less likely to develop silent infarcts or stroke, and individuals who ate fish just once a week were 13 percent less likely to do so, according to a report on the research. Regular consumers of fish also showed fewer signs of negative changes to their brains' white matter, a factor often associated with memory decline. Fried fish did not confer the same protective effects as broiled or baked fish, the researchers found

Another study suggests that fish oil supplements can improve memory performance in older adults with mild memory complaints (See Box 6-1). However, although the supplements appear to improve brain health and memory performance in early memory decline, so far no human studies have found that these benefits have an effect on Alzheimer's progression.

Omega-3 fatty acids may produce their beneficial effect on memory by boosting the production of a protein known to destroy the beta-amyloid plaques associated with AD. Some research suggests the omega-3 fatty acid docosahexaenoic acid (DHA) may increase the production of a specific protein in the brain that has been shown to destroy beta-amyloid plaques. The plaques are a key characteristic of Alzheimer's disease (AD) and are thought to be toxic to brain cells. Building on earlier research that demonstrated that individuals with AD have low brain levels of a protein called LR11 that is thought to prevent the build-up of beta-amyloid plaque, the scientists tested whether DHA might affect LR11 levels. The researchers administered fish oil or DHA directly to rat neurons and human neurons grown in the laboratory. They also included it in the diets of living rats and mice bred to develop AD to observe the effects on LR11 levels. The research revealed that even low doses of DHA led to a significant increase in levels of plaque-destroying LR11 in cell cultures and in living animals. The study's authors recommended undertaking large-scale clinical trials to determine whether fish oil or DHA can be used at early stages of AD to help slow or prevent disease progression.

Several other supplements have been considered as possibly having beneficial effects on memory and slowing Alzheimer's disease progression, but the few small trials conducted to measure their effects have been largely inconclusive, and research continues. Among the supplements with possible—but as yet unproven—memory effects are vincpocetine (derived from the leaves of the common periwinkle) and acetyl-L-carnitine (a vitamin-like substance). ■

NEW FINDING

Box 6-1: Fish oil supplements may improve memory

A study involving older adults with mild memory complaints who took omega-3 pills for six months suggests that the fish oil supplements can help improve memory performance. Researchers divided into two groups 485 healthy participants 55 and older with memory problems associated with age-related memory decline (such as forgetting names or appointments). One group took 900 mg per day of docosahexanoic acid (DHA, an omega-3 fatty acid found in abundant quantities algae and oils from cold-water fish) and the second group received an inactive placebo. Both groups of participants were given memory tests at the beginning and end of the six-month study, and their blood levels of DHA were assessed. By the end of the study, the participants who took DHA had doubled their blood levels of DHA, and experienced twice the reduction in number of errors on memory tests as participants who took placebo—a benefit roughly equivalent to having the memory skills of a person three years younger. The higher a participant's DHA levels, the better his or her performance on memory tests were, according to a report on the study published online May 4, 2010 in *Alzheimer's & Dementia: The Journal of the Alzheimer's Association.*

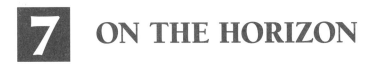

7 ON THE HORIZON

Although drugs currently available can ease some of the symptoms of Alzheimer's, they have had only limited success, and are often accompanied by serious side effects. Researchers are working on a number of new drugs, many of which hold great promise and hope for people with Alzheimer's.

Drugs in the pipeline

The goal of the next generation of Alzheimer's disease drugs will be to slow, prevent, or perhaps even reverse the course of memory loss. Many of the drugs in the pharmaceutical pipeline are targeting the root causes of Alzheimer's disease, specifically the factors that lead to the development of tangles inside the brain's neurons that kill the nerve cells, or the formation of sticky beta-amyloid plaques that also ultimately result in cell death. Researchers are attempting to modify the outcome of Alzheimer's disease by directly affecting the mechanisms that ultimately destroy memory and brain function.

"We know much more about the workings of the brain now than we did just 10 or 20 years ago," says Dr. Falk. "These discoveries, along with other findings about the brain that have resulted from advances in molecular biology, bioengineering, genetics and other fields, have opened up whole new avenues of research, leading to new possibilities for the treatment of memory disorders and dementia."

The U.S. Food and Drug Administration (FDA) requires that before new drugs are made available to the public, they undergo a highly structured and careful evaluation process to test their effectiveness and potential risks. Many promising new drugs in initial stages of development are in phase II trials designed to assess safety and efficacy of medications in the target population and to determine the correct dosages. Drugs in a later stage of development are assessed in phase III trials, which involve larger groups of subjects, typically last a year or more, and are designed to provide a more thorough understanding of the drug's benefits and side effects.

"Generally speaking, it's best to take a conservative approach when considering potential new therapies," cautions Dr. Falk. "Although many new approaches may do well in animal research or early human trials, they may later prove to be ineffective or to cause undesirable side effects. Even when a drug shows promise, it may be years before it is available in clinical practice. Still, the search for new therapies helps move us in the right direction."

By attacking the root causes of Alzheimer's disease, new drugs under development aim to halt the progressive slide to deepening memory loss, and perhaps even reverse damage that has already occurred. Below are some of the most promising treatments for Alzheimer's currently being investigated, some of which—if they are successful in all stages of human trials—could be available within the next few years.

Dimebon

The drug dimebon (brand name Dimebon), which has been used as an antihistamine in Russia for many years, appeared in a phase II trial in Russia to help protect against the death of brain cells in neurodegenerative diseases such as Alzheimer's. Dimebon is thought to target cellular power generators, called mitochondria, in the brain. In preclinical tests, the drug appeared to help protect mitochondria against pathological changes that can trigger brain cell death, working in part by reducing excessive amounts of a key neurotransmitter, glutamate, in fluids that surround brain cells.

Phase II trials suggested that the medication was associated with significant improvements compared to placebo in all the key aspects of Alzheimer's, including thinking, memory, behavior and overall function. In a double-blind, placebo-controlled trial involving 183 individuals with mild to moderate AD, researchers reported that study participants who took Dimebon appeared to stabilize and improve, while participants who took placebo experienced cognitive decline. Over one year, Dimebon was associated with significant improvement in measures of cognition, such as memory, orientation, and language, researchers reported. The drug also stabilized behavioral symptoms such as depression, hallucinations, and irritability. Benefits continued to increase over time and were larger at the end of one year than they had been at six months, according to a report presented published a few years ago in *The Lancet*. Side effects of the drug were minor.

A longer confirmatory phase III trial was launched with high hopes. But in March 2010, Medivation, the manufacturer of Dimebon and co-sponsor Pfizer Inc. released data from the trial that revealed that Dimebon did not have any significant effect on AD progression (see Box 7-1) and chances of Dimebon obtaining FDA approval in the next year or so seem increasingly remote.

Methylthioninium chloride (Rember)

An investigation involving the experimental drug methylthioninium chloride (Rember) as a treatment for mild to moderate Alzheimer's disease stirred excitement at the 2008 Alzheimer's Association's International Conference on Alzheimer's Disease in Chicago, when the researchers announced that the compound appeared to stabilize disease progression in patients with mild and moderate Alzheimer's. The drug is believed to attack AD by dissolving tangles of tau protein inside brain cells and preventing their accumulation, and researchers reported that it safely slowed cognitive decline by as much as 81 percent over a period of 19 months in 321 patients with mild to moderate AD. In brain scans conducted after a 24-week, Phase II trial, researchers reported that the drug produced significantly better blood flow to brain regions associated with memory compared to placebo, an indication of increased brain activity. Results suggest the drug was helping to dissolve destructive tau protein filaments (neurofibrillary tangles) that accumulate within neurons. Cognitive measures of participants who continued using the drug over 19 months were not significantly different from measures taken at the outset of the study, but study participants not taking the drug experienced significant decline over the same period.

Unfortunately, since the hopeful announcements that accompanied the 2008 release of the Phase II Rember study results, there has been little progress—or information about—Rember, and the manufacturer's plans for further trials for the drug are not clear at this time.

Davunetide

Another approach, a new drug called davunetide intranasal (AL-108), targets a key characteristic of AD, abnormal changes in a protein called tau that result in damaging neurofibrillary tangles inside brain cells. Davunetide contains fragments of a protein responsible for protecting nerve cells against severe oxidative stress and toxicity, and helps block the formation of neurofibrillary tangles. In a Phase II trial involving 144 men and women ages 55 to 85 with mild cognitive impairment (considered an early form of AD), researchers compared a nasal spray containing davunetide with placebo. After 16 weeks, study participants who received the drug showed a 62.4 percent improvement on tests of memory performance, with no side effects. The changes were "statistically significant, dose-dependent and durable," study authors said in a presentation at the July 2008 Alzheimer's Association's International Conference on Alzheimer's Disease in Chicago.

On March 15, 2009, researchers reported on an animal study of the drug at the 9th International Conference for Alzheimer's Disease and Parkinson's Disease. Their investigation involved treating mice bred to develop mutations of the tau gene with davunetide and comparing them to similar animals who did not receive the drug. After five months, mice treated daily with the drug demonstrated increased learning and memory performance compared with controls. Comparison of the brains of treated mice with untreated mice after 10 months showed that treated mice had significantly lower levels of abnormal tau tangles than untreated mice.

The developer of davunetide, Allon Therapeutics, announced on March 11, 2010, that it had completed a Phase 1 clinical trial that broadened the demonstrated safety and dose range of davunetide. The drug, which has been shown to be effective and safe in humans in daily doses of 5 mg and 30 mg, was evaluated for safety at doses up to 60 mg per day in the latest trial.

Allon Therapeutics is now planning to conduct a longer Phase II trial involving human patients.

Immunoglobulins

Immunoglobulins, or antibodies, are gamma globulin proteins in the blood that are used by the immune system to hunt down and eliminate bacteria, viruses and other invaders. Two blood products containing immunoglobulins are being investigated for their effects on AD.

One product, immunoglobulin M (IgM), has shown promise in animal research. Scientists gave mice bred to develop an animal version of AD a single intravenous dose of IgM, with promising results. The antibodies seemed to bind with beta-amyloid proteins in the brain, preventing them from developing into sticky plaque and reversing cognitive impairment similar to that seen in humans with AD, the researchers reported.

Another product, intravenous immunoglobulin (IVIg), is already used in humans to treat disorders of the immune system, but also may be beneficial for people with Alzheimer's. IVIg contains antibodies against the beta-amyloid protein that promotes the formation of plaques in the brain characteristic of Alzheimer's disease (AD).

Research suggests that natural antibodies contained in IVIg bind to and eliminate clusters of beta-amyloid peptide molecules that are thought to be involved in AD causation. People with mild-to-moderate Alzheimer's disease who were treated with the antibodies in small preliminary studies showed improvement on cognitive tests. Measures of beta-amyloid levels in the patients' cerebrospinal fluid (an indication of beta-amyloid elimination) rose significantly after the first six months, returned to original levels when treatment was discontinued, then remained stable during subsequent IVIg treatment.

In April 2010, researchers announced that treatment with a formulation of immunoglobulin called Gammagard for 18 months significantly reduced brain atrophy and helped preserve thinking abilities in a group of people with mild to moderate Alzheimer's disease (see Box 7-2).

Rosiglitazone (Avandia)

A drug commonly used to treat type 2 diabetes was investigated as a possible treatment for Alzheimer's disease, with disappointing results. The drug, rosiglitazone

(Avandia), helps diabetes patients by enabling their cells to use the hormone insulin more efficiently, and it was hoped the drug might bolster response to insulin and block the action of toxic proteins that attack brain cells in Alzheimer's disease. Avandia carried risks, however, and the manufacturer had been instructed by the FDA to include a warning label on drug packaging emphasizing that the medication may increase the risk of heart attacks. In 2010, the FDA placed strict requirements on who could have access to Avandia, while the drug continues to be investigated.

In July 2009, the manufacturer of Avandia, GlaxoSmithKline Plc, announced that Avandia had failed to provide benefit in a large six-month study of 553 people with mild to moderate Alzheimer's disease. At that time, the company ended the study, along with two other trials of the drug.

Alzheimer's vaccine

Another method for targeting Alzheimer's comes in the form of a vaccine that uses antibodies from the body's own immune system to attack and destroy beta-amyloid and clear out plaques in the brain, or to eliminate clumps of tau protein (neurofibrillary tangles) in the brain that kill neurons responsible for memory.

A pathological form of tau, which tends to collect inside cells in the memory centers of the brains of individuals with AD, is toxic to neurons and causes degeneration and death of brain cells. Several years ago, animal research revealed that a vaccine could successfully prompt the body to attack abnormal tau proteins.

Researchers injected mice genetically engineered to develop the fibrous tangles with a vaccine containing fragments of abnormal tau, then looked to see whether the immune system would mount a defense against the destructive proteins. Compared to similar mice that were not immunized, animals that received the vaccine performed better in tests of motor skills and were more apt to remain cognitively normal. Examinations of their brains showed less evidence of tau protein tangles, the researchers said. The study findings—which suggest that antibodies generated by the body in response to a tau vaccine are absorbed by ailing cells, where they target and clear the destructive tangles—may lead to promising therapies in humans.

In 2002, a first attempt at a vaccine-based therapy targeting beta-amyloid plaque in humans was halted when about six percent of the patients in the study developed dangerous brain inflammation believed to be caused by the vaccine agent. However, when researchers followed up with study participants four-and-a-half years after immunization, people who had developed antibodies to beta-amyloid experienced a slower cognitive decline than patients given a placebo, and there were no additional cases of brain inflammation, according to the vaccine's developer, the Irish pharmaceutical company Elan Corporation.

Because of the promising aspects of the therapy, research continued in an effort to develop a safer version of the vaccine. In January 2007, scientists reported some success in studies using a patch version of the reformulated vaccine on mice. The mice given the patch vaccine developed high levels of antibodies to beta-amyloid, as well as evidence that beta-amyloid proteins were being removed from their brains, researchers reported in the *Proceedings of the National Academy of Sciences.*

Pfizer, Johnson & Johnson and Elan now have a newer version of the vaccine in the works—an antibody called bapineuzumab that is designed to attack and eliminate beta-amyloid plaque. In Phase II trials, the drug did not significantly slow Alzheimer's progression in the overall study population, but there were indications that the drug might slow decline in individuals with AD who do not have the ApoE4 genetic mutation that increases risk for the disease (about one-third of all Alzheimer's patients). Phase III trials of the drug are now underway, with results expected in 2012.

A recent study involving bapineuzumab—intended to test a new scanning technique designed to measure the efficacy of Alzheimer therapies—has shed additional light on the drug. The imaging study found that bapineuzumab reduced amyloid plaque levels by 25 percent, but found no effect on patients' cognitive abilities (see Box 7-3).

Meanwhile, a preliminary human trial involving a vaccine developed by Eli Lilly and Company that targets beta-amyloid has shown promising preliminary results. The drug, called solanezumab (LY2061430), is designed to bind with beta-amyloid protein and help dissolve it and eliminate it from the body. The plaques are associated with AD and have long been thought to be linked to brain cell death. The study involved 53 individuals with mild to moderate AD. Half of participants received the solanezumab vaccine intravenously, and half received placebo. In the three-month trial, levels of beta-amyloid in the blood and spinal fluid increased, suggesting that solanezumab was successfully dissolving beta-amyloid plaques present in the brain. However, the trial was too brief to demonstrate improvements in memory. Solanezumab caused no significant side effects in patients, according to researchers.

A longer, Phase III study involving 1,000 people is currently underway. The 19-month trial is expected to be completed in 2012.

There is research that suggests the elimination of plaque may not restore cognitive function. A study comparing canines treated with a vaccine designed to produce antibodies against beta-amyloid with similar dogs that were not immunized. Researchers found little difference between vaccinated dogs and unvacci-

---

NEW FINDING

Box 7-3: New biomarker measures effectiveness of AD drug bapineuzumab

Researchers used a new biomarker and scanning technique to measure the effects of the investigational Alzheimer's disease (AD) drug bapineuzumab, proving the usefulness of the technique in evaluating AD treatment. Their findings suggest that the drug reduced levels of amyloid plaque by 25 percent over 78 weeks. Researchers used a biomarker tracker called carbon 11-labeled Pittsburgh compound B (C-PIB) along with positron emission tomography (PET) scans to compare 20 AD patients treated with bapineuzumab with eight patients who received an inactive placebo. Participants were administered one-hour intravenous infusions every 13 weeks for up to six infusions. PET scans were administered at the outset of the study, and at 20, 45 and 78 weeks. Participants also underwent laboratory tests, magnetic resonance imaging, and tests of cognition. At the end of the study, participants given bapineuzumab demonstrated a 25 percent reduction in beta-amyloid plaque compared to participants given placebo, results suggests bapineuzumab increases the clearance of plaque from the brain. However, the study, published online March 1, 2010 in *Lancet Neurology*, did not detect any Improvement in thinking or reasoning among study participants. Researchers suggested there might have been greater differences between drug and placebo groups if treatment was extended over a longer time. Bapineuzumab is now in late-stage clinical trials.

An animal study that explored the role of free-floating bits of toxic beta-amyloid protein called oligomers in Alzheimer's disease (AD) suggests that it may be these proteins, and not beta-amyloid plaque, that cause the death of brain cells. Plaque has long been considered a major cause of AD, and a number of investigational drugs target these sticky masses that form inside the brain. Researchers genetically engineered mice to form only oligomers, but not brain plaque. In tests of memory and thinking, the genetically engineered mice showed the same evidence of cognitive problems as a control group of mice that had both plaque and oligomers. Researchers then treated the oligomer mice with a gene that cause them to form plaque. The addition of plaque did not make the oligomer-induced memory problems any worse, according to researchers, who published their investigation in the April 2010 issue of *Annals of Neurology*. The findings suggest that it may be beta-amyloid oligomers, and not plaque, that cause the destruction associated with AD, and that drugs currently under development that aim to improve symptoms of AD by eliminating plaque may be missing their target.

nated dogs in behavioral tests that measured cognitive decline, even though autopsies later showed that in immunized animals, plaques had been eliminated from brain regions involved with learning and memory. The study authors reported that despite the absence of plaques, damaged neurons remained, providing a possible explanation for the behavioral-test results.

The findings seem to support a new theory of Alzheimer's causation that suggests that free-floating bits of beta-amyloid rather than sticky beta-amyloid plaque may be behind the death of brain cells in AD. The theory has raised questions about the premise behind vaccines designed to eliminate plaque. If plaque is not the primary source of the toxicity that creates Alzheimer's damage, but rather represents an effort by the body to protect brain cells by binding and disabling the actual toxic agent—free-floating beta-amyloid—then plaque-fighting AD vaccines are missing the target. What's more, it is not clear if the vaccines affect free-floating beta-amyloid at all, since it is not possible to track the accumulation of these small proteins with brain scanning technology, as can be done with plaque, and research suggests that lowering levels of plaque does not result in improvement of AD symptoms (see Box 7-4).

Gene therapy

Researchers are working hard to find ways to use genetic therapies in the prevention and treatment of Alzheimer's disease, and there have been a number of encouraging findings.

In 2004, a small initial test using gene therapy suggested that inserting cells genetically altered to produce growth factors into the brains of people with Alzheimer's may slow the destruction of brain cells. Researchers took skin cells from Alzheimer's patients and genetically modified them to release a protein called nerve growth factor (NGF), which helps prevent brain cell death and stimulates cell function in healthy brains. The altered cells then were surgically implanted into a deep brain region in the patients where cell degeneration associated with AD typically occurs. PET scans done after the procedure showed an increase in brain metabolic activity and cognitive tests showed a 50 percent reduction in annual rates of decline compared to rates before the procedure.

In another study, researchers used genetic engineering in mice to target an immune molecule called transforming growth factor or TGF-beta, which helps activate the immune system in response to injury. People with AD have higher levels of this molecule in their bodies. The researchers blocked TGF-beta in the peripheral immune system, outside the brain, causing the release of peripheral cells called macrophages that target and destroy foreign material in the body. Those macrophages were able to cross the blood-brain barrier to envelop and destroy beta-amyloid within the brain of the mice, eliminating up to 90 percent of the beta-amyloid plaques clogging their brain tissue, according to a report published online May, 2008 in the journal *Nature Medicine*. The mice who received the treatment showed improved performance on tests of memory. The findings offer the possibility of developing drugs for humans that can be introduced into the bloodstream to cause peripheral immune cells to target beta-amyloid plaques in the brain.

These animal studies set the stage for the utilization of genetic therapies in humans with AD. The surgery necessary to implant cells directly into the brain has significant risks, and gene therapy techniques that involve injecting Alzheimer's patients with genetically modified viruses also may raise safety concerns for humans. Nevertheless, the first study testing the effectiveness of gene therapy for people with AD began enrolling participants in 2010 (see Box 7-5).

Histone deacetylase (HDAC) inhibitor

Drugs called histone deacetylase (HADC) inhibitors—which reduce the effect of certain genes in the brain that are involved in impaired learning—are offering new promise in the effort to fight age-related memory decline and Alzheimer's. The drugs, which are already in development for use in people with certain cancers, have shown significant brain benefits in animal studies, and human studies may be initiated soon.

The HDAC inhibitor compound was formulated after researchers at the Massachusetts Institute of Technology (MIT) tested the effects of HDAC inhibitors on mice whose brains were genetically engineered to develop memory problems. The researchers had taught the mice how to get through a maze to find food before inducing memory loss. After taking the drug, the mice with memory loss developed new cell dendrites and synapses (cell projections involved in the transmission of nerve impulses), and their ability to navigate through the maze improved significantly. Interestingly, impaired mice that were placed in an enriched environment where they had access to toys and exercise wheels also did better on the maze test. The research suggests that people with dementia might not completely lose their memories, but that the memories might be stored away somewhere that is inaccessible.

In another study using mice bred to develop Alzheimer's disease (AD), researchers identified a gene—HADC2—and its associated protein that could be targeted by drugs to help reverse the effects of AD and improve cognitive function. Their experiments showed that treatment with HADC inhibitors caused mice to regain long-term memories and the ability to learn new tasks, according to a report in the

May 7, 2009 issue of *Nature*. On May 7, 2010, researchers published a study in the journal *Science* reporting that changes in the way genes are expressed in older mice are associated with impaired memory and learning, and that HADC inhibitor drugs could reverse these changes.

Several studies using mice and dogs have already established the safety of HADC inhibitor drugs; the next step involves clinical trials in humans to assess whether HDAC inhibitors can safely and effectively improve cognition and possibly reverse memory loss. "We have finished the first phase—the pre-clinical phase—and now it's time for the pharmaceutical industry to really try and drive it into application," said a co-author of the *Science* study.

Intranasal Insulin

An insulin spray applied through the nose has shown promise in the treatment of people with AD, according to a small preliminary study. A group of 104 adults with MCI and AD received either two doses of 20 or 40 international units of intranasal insulin or two doses of placebo every day for four months. All participants underwent testing at the outset of the study, and again at two and four months. Smaller groups of participants had lumbar punctures or brain scans to ascertain biomarker profiles and levels of brain activity. Participants who received placebo showed evidence of cognitive decline, whereas participants who received insulin preserved or improved memory and functioning, according to a report presented July 14, 2010, at the International Conference on Alzheimer's Disease. Study participants who received insulin also showed evidence of improvement in brain activity and biomarker profiles. Insulin receptors are widely distributed in the brain, where the hormone is thought to help regulate beta-amyloid proteins associated with AD and promote the functioning of synaptic connections among nerve cells. The study authors say further trials are needed before insulin sprays can be used in clinical settings.

Promising preliminary findings

A number of studies in animals suggest new possibilities for Alzheimer's therapies. Among the more interesting potential treatments currently being explored are:

- Brain-Derived Neurotrophic Factor (BDNF): Researchers used injections of this naturally occurring brain protein to halt or reverse the process of cell degeneration and cell death in aged rats and in mice bred to have Alzheimer's symptoms. The injections into the brains of the lab animals stimulated treated animals to begin producing more BDNF on their own, and led to long-term improvements in performance on tests of memory and cognitive skills. Untreated animals continued to decline, according to a report in the February 8, 2009 issue of *Nature Medicine*. "BDNF treatment can potentially provide long-lasting protection by slowing, or even stopping, disease progression in the cortical regions that receive treatment," the lead author said.

- **Granulocyte-colony stimulating factor (GCSF)**: Another growth factor, GCSF stimulates blood stem cells production in the bone marry. In mice bred to develop Alzheimer's disease, the growth factor reverses memory impairment and significantly reduces brain levels of beta-amyloid plaque, according to a report in the August 2009 online issue of *Neuroscience*. Examination of the animals' brains also revealed the development of new nerve cells and nerve cell connections.

- **Sodium phenylbutyrate**: Mice bred to have symptoms of an Alzheimer's-like disease showed improvements in learning and memory after being treated with sodium phenylbutyrate, a drug currently widely used to treat a hereditary metabolic disorder in humans. The medication targets the deterioration of connections among neurons, helping the brain to assimilate and store new memories, according the lead author of the study. The research was published in the February 2009 issue of the journal *Neuropsychopharmacology*.

- **Liver treatment**: Laboratory experiments involving rats have revealed a potentially effective means of removing neuron-damaging beta-amyloid proteins—a hallmark of Alzheimer's disease—from the brain. Researchers decreased the ability of the liver to clear beta-amyloid in the bloodstream to determine whether levels of the protein in the bloodstream were linked to levels in the brain. They observed that the increase of beta-amyloid in the bloodstream was accompanied by a dramatic decrease in the clearance of the toxic proteins from the brain. The results suggest that the liver's role in clearing beta-amyloid from the blood leads, in turn, to reducing accumulation of beta-amyloid in the brain, and that finding ways to boost the liver's ability to clear beta-amyloid in the blood might be an effective avenue for treating the elevated brain levels of beta-amyloid characteristic of Alzheimer's disease. A report o n the study was published in the February 2009 *Journal of Alzheimer's Disease*.

- **The vascular drug hydroxyfasudil (Fasudil)**: Researchers injected hydroxyfasudil (a drug used in humans to treat vascular problems by dilating blood vessels in the brain) into middle-aged male rats. Memory testing showed that rats given a high dose of the drug learned and remembered more information and those given a low dose. Rats in both drug groups performed significantly better on tests of memory and learning than a group of rats that received only an inactive saline solution. "The collected findings and the relative safety of Fasudil support its potential…as a cognitive enhancer in humans who have age- or neurodegenerative-related memory dysfunction," the researchers concluded in a report in the February 2009 issue of *Behavioral Neuroscience.*

◼ Nerve cell transplants: Researchers report that nerve cells transplanted into brain memory regions of rats that had suffered injury to those regions triggered the full recovery of the animals' ability to learn and remember information. According to a study published in the December 2009 issue of *Behavioral Neuroscience*, memory tests revealed that, compared to injured rats that did not receive injections of nerve cells and did not recover memory function, rats that underwent nerve-cell transplants had completely recovered from their brain injuries and performed as well as healthy rats. Examination of the animals' brains showed that in the transplant rats, transplanted cells had localized to an area of the hippocampus (a key memory region that shrinks under the onslaught of Alzheimer's disease) called the dentate gyrus. There, the cells apparently increased the secretion of growth factors that promote the growth and survival of cells that give rise to new neurons. For example, levels of brain-derived neurotrophic factor (BDNF) were three times higher in transplant rats. The findings may ultimately lead to therapies that can reverse the effects of aging or dementia.

◼ Targeting the PXR receptor: A study published in the May 2010 issue of *Molecular Pharmacology* describes a novel approach to slowing Alzheimer's disease (AD) by targeting a specific receptor in the blood-brain barrier. The blood-brain barrier protects the brain by isolating it from the bloodstream, preventing the entry of toxic chemicals, and removing toxic proteins and metabolites from the brain. Working with laboratory mice bred to produce the toxic human beta-amyloid protein associated with AD, researchers used a steroid-like chemical to activate a brain receptor known as the pregnane Xreceptor, or PXR. Activationof the receptor, in turn, increased the expression of a blood-brain barrier protein called P-glycoprotein, whic h plays an important role in clearing beta-amyloid from the brain. The procedure reduced the accumulation of beta-amyloid in the brains of the experimental mice to levels seen in healthy mice, the researchers reported. "This study may provide the experimental basis for new strategies that can be used to treat Alzheimer's patients," the lead author said. ◼

8 HELPING YOURSELF

While new drugs under development hold promise that in the future we will find ways of mitigating and perhaps even reversing the effects of Alzheimer's disease and other forms of dementia, none of these medications is going to be available for several years. In the meantime, there is much you can do to protect your brain and memory.

"All people experience brain changes as they get older—they are an inevitable part of aging," explains Dr. Blacker. "Many of these changes are perfectly normal. They vary from person to person—some people will have more changes, some will have fewer—and they may affect different parts of a person's cognitive capacities to varying degrees.

"The best way to protect your memory is to keep your brain as healthy as possible for as long as possible. Taking care of your brain by avoiding cardiovascular disease and diabetes, specifically through exercise and proper nutrition, controlling weight, and maintaining healthy cholesterol and blood pressure levels can improve your chances of keeping your memory sharp well into old age."

Ways to lower your dementia risk
Eat brain-healthy foods

A healthy diet is essential to maintaining your brain in peak condition. Brain cells need a rich and varied supply of vitamins and nutrients to grow and function properly, and to resist and repair damage (see Box 8-1 on the following page). Important elements supplied by foods help protect your brain from free radicals (unstable molecules that cause injury to brain cells through a process called oxidation) that play a role in Alzheimer's disease and other disorders. The right foods help boost mental energy, improve concentration, and strengthen communication among brain cells. A healthy diet also helps lower your risk for cardiovascular disease: High blood pressure, hardening of the arteries, stroke, and disease of the small blood vessels of the brain all can contribute to memory decline.

What kind of diet will give your brain a boost? A menu that's high in nutrients and relatively low in fat is best for brain health. Eating four to six small meals throughout the day, rather than three big ones, will help provide your brain with a steady supply of fuel and make you feel more alert. Drink a minimum of eight glasses of water each day: Research on the effects of dehydration on cognitive function suggests that dehydration that results in the loss of as little as one percent of body weight can have a negative effect on mental performance.

Eat plenty of fresh fruits and vegetables such as spinach, strawberries, blueberries, and carrots, which are high in brain-protecting antioxidants. Add whole-grain products, such as bread, cereal, pasta, and brown rice, for complex carbohydrates that provide healthy levels of the brain fuel glucose to give your brain energy and improve memory function. Research suggests that glucose—or sugar—may improve episodic memory, a form of memory involving recollections of events. Investigators administered memory tests to 48 older adults, then divided the study participants into two groups. One group was given a sweet-flavored drink containing glucose; the second group received a sweet-flavored placebo that contained no glucose. In memory tests following consumption of the sweet drinks, subjects given glucose experienced significant improvement on tasks involving episodic memory, while subjects given placebo showed no improvement—an indication of the importance of adequate supplies of glucose to memory functioning.

Another study suggests that improving the way your body metabolizes sugar through a healthy diet, exercise, or medication can help stave off memory changes associated with aging. High blood sugar levels can directly affect the hippocampus, a brain region responsible for memory and learning. Researchers used functional magnetic resonance imaging (fMRI) to map the hippocampus in 240 older adults without apparent memory problems. The scientists looked at changes that frequently accompany normal aging—such as increasing body mass index and rising levels of cholesterol, insulin and blood sugar—to determine which factors

BOX 8-1: 11 VITAMINS FOR A HEALTHY BRAIN

These 11 nutritional powerhouses help ensure that your brain is working at maximum capacity. Foods, which provide additional important nutrients, are the best source, but a daily multivitamin is a good alternative. Follow these guidelines to ensure that you're getting enough of these brain-boosting vitamins: (note: mcg = micrograms; mg = miligrams; IU = international unit)

VITAMIN	WHAT IT DOES	RECOMMENDED DAILY ALLOWANCE (RDA)	SOURCES
Vitamin A	Protects the brain cells from unstable molecules called free radicals that can cause damage	women: 800 mcg men: 1,000 mcg	Liver, carrots, dark-colored fruits, leafy vegetables
Vitamin B1 (Thiamin)	Keeps the nervous system healthy	women: 1 mg; men: 1.2 mg	Whole-grain or fortified breads, cereals
Vitamin B2 (Riboflavin)	Enhances energy production in the brain cells	women: 1.2 mg; men: 1.4 mg	Milk, organ meats, fortified breads, cereals
Vitamin B3 (Niacin)	Needed for energy metabolism	women: 13 mg men: 15 mg	Meat, fish, poultry, whole-grain bread, fortified cereals
Vitamin B5 (Pantothenic acid)	Helps transmit nerve impulses; important for adrenal cortex function.	5 mg	Chicken, beef, potatoes, oats, cereals, tomato products, egg yolk, broccoli
Vitamin B6 (Pyridoxine)	Needed for production of the brain chemicals serotonin, dopamine, norepinephrine, adrenaline	women: 1.6 mg men: 2 mg	Fortified cereals, organ meats
Vitamin B9 (Folic acid)	Needed for metabolism of fatty acids in the brain; important in neurotransmitter production like B12	women: 180 mcg men: 200 mcg	Dark leafy greens, enriched and whole-grain bread products, fortified cereals
Vitamin B12	Helps produce the brain chemicals serotonin, norepinephrine and dopamine	2 mcg	Meat, fish, poultry, fortified cereals
Vitamin C	Acts as an antioxidant to protect the brain cells from damage	60 mg	Citrus fruits, blueberries, tomatoes, spinach, potatoes, Brussels sprouts, strawberries
Vitamin D	Needed for the absorption of calcium and phosphorous	10 mcg or 400 IU	Fish liver oils, fatty fish, fortified dairy products, cereals
Vitamin E	Might protect nerve cells from damage	women: 8 mg men: 10 mg	Vegetable oils, unprocessed cereal grains, nuts, fruits, vegetables, meats

were most closely associated with deterioration of key areas of the hippocampus, a brain region essential to learning and memory.

The researchers found that the only factor closely correlated to decreasing activity in the dentate gyrus, a sub-region associated with age-related memory decline, was increased levels of blood glucose, suggesting the blood sugar abnormalities were implicated in hippocampal dysfunction. The study's authors concluded that because blood sugar levels rise with age, even people without diabetes would benefit from strategies such as exercise, changes in diet, or medication that can improve blood sugar levels and possibly delay age-associated cognitive decline. "Improving glucose metabolism could be a clinically viable approach for improving the cognitive slide that occurs in many of us as we age," the lead author of the study said.

Low-fat dairy foods, nuts, seeds, and beans, and occasional servings of eggs, poultry, and lean meats provide protein that helps keep your mind alert, along with vitamins and other nutrients that promote the growth of new brain cells and support brain functioning (see Box 8-2). Healthy fats such as monounsaturated canola and olive oils, which can help lower levels of LDL ("bad") cholesterol, and polyunsaturated oils such as those derived from corn, cottonseeds, and sunflower seeds, are essential to the absorption of certain vitamins and provide energy that heightens alertness.

One type of polyunsaturated fat—omega-3 fatty acids—is especially important to brain health. Research is finding that these fatty acids, which are most commonly found in cold-water fish, play a key role in cognitive function. Getting too little of this nutrient in your diet may put you at risk for a number of diseases and events, including Alzheimer's and stroke. To boost your omega-3 levels, eat salmon, sardines, mackerel, tuna, or shrimp at least twice a week. Other good sources are flaxseed, dark-green leafy vegetables and fish-oil supplements.

Caring for your brain requires not only adding nutritious foods to your diet, but avoiding unhealthy foods as well. Reduce or eliminate saturated fats such as butter and lard, and trans fats (hydrogenated or partially hydrogenated oils) that are found in many commercially prepared fried foods, processed foods, and snack foods. These unhealthy fats can raise levels of artery-clogging LDL cholesterol. Go easy on simple carbohydrates such as processed white rice and flour, and refined sugars, as these foods can increase your risk of developing insulin resistance, a condition that may be a contributing factor in the development of AD.

There are a number of healthy eating plans for you to choose from, including the National Heart, Lung and Blood Institute's Dietary Approaches to Stop Hypertension (DASH) diet and the U.S. Department of Agriculture's Mypyramid.gov.

NEW FINDING

Box 8-2: Dietary magnesium boosts short- and long-term memory

Eat your beans and greens. Both are loaded with magnesium, a mineral that helps regulate a key brain receptor important for learning and memory. According to a study published in the January 28, 2010 issue of *Neuron*, rats fed a magnesium compound showed significant gains in short-and long-term memory, working memory, and ability to learn, and older rats fed the compound performed better on a range of learning tests. The magnesium supplement increased and strengthened the connections among brain cells in the hippocampus, a key memory region of the brain. Experts say only 32 percent of Americans get the recommended daily allowance of magnesium, which is found naturally in dark leafy vegetables, nuts, legumes, tofu, and whole grains.

The Mediterranean Diet (see Box 8-3)—which limits meat and dairy products and emphasizes fruits and vegetables, fish, and monounsaturated fats such as olive and canola oils—is an example of a diet plan that benefits the brain. It is based on the dietary patterns in Mediterranean countries in which life expectancy is high and incidence of chronic disease is low.

In addition to lowering risk for heart disease and cancer, Mediterranean-style diets are associated with reduced risk for developing mild cognitive impairment (MCI), a transitional stage between normal cognition and dementia/Alzheimer's disease. Researchers compared the diets of 1,393 healthy older adults with the diets of 482 people with MCI, and followed both groups for an average of 4.5 years. They found that people who adhered most closely to a Mediterranean-style diet—characterized by plenty of vegetables, fish, fruits, nuts, and grains, and low amounts of saturated fat, meat, dairy products and alcohol—were 28 percent less likely than people who did not adhere to the Mediterranean-style diet to develop MCI. Those who followed an intermediate Mediterranean-style diet were 17 percent less likely to develop MCI, according to a report on the study published in the February 2009 *Archives of Neurology*. Among people who had MCI at the outset of the study, adherence to the diet was associated with a lower risk of progressing to dementia. Of this group, 106 individuals developed dementia; risk for progression to dementia was 48 percent lower in subjects who adhered most closely to the Mediterranean-style diet, and 45 percent lower among those with intermediate adherence compared to individuals with the lowest adherence scores. Study authors theorized that the Mediterranean diet may help improve blood vessel health, lower blood-sugar and cholesterol levels, and reduce inflammation, all factors that have been linked to greater risk for MCI. Components of the diet—such as fish and the replacement of saturated fats with polyunsaturated fatty acids such as olive or canola oil—may also contribute to the beneficial effects.

In a major study conducted several years ago by researchers at Columbia University, 2,258 older adults in New York City were asked to follow the Mediterranean Diet for four years. At the end of the study period, researchers found that those participants who adhered most closely to the diet were 40 percent less likely than those who failed to adhere to the diet to develop Alzheimer's disease. Although further research is needed, the study suggests that the Mediterranean Diet can help protect the brain from AD. The researchers believe that the combination of foods, rather than any single component of the diet, may be responsible for the protective effects.

BOX 8-3

The traditional healthy Mediterranean Diet Pyramid

The Mediterranean Diet Pyramid is based on an overall pattern of healthy eating. Only general amounts are given for foods in the pyramid, since specific amounts may vary substantially from country to country. The diet characteristically includes the following: Plenty of foods from plant sources, such as breads and grains, potatoes, fruits and vegetables, seeds, beans, and nuts; olive oil as the principal source of fat, with limited intake of saturated fat; low to moderate amounts of (preferably low-fat) cheese or yogurt each day; up to four eggs a week; low to moderate amounts of fish and poultry each week; sweet desserts several times a week; lean red meat once or twice a month (maximum of 12 to 16 ounces total); and moderate amounts of wine (up to two glasses a day for men, one glass a day for women), along with six to eight glasses of water daily. Regular physical activity is also associated with a healthful Mediterranean lifestyle.

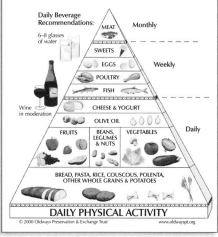

Watch your waistline

While a definitive link between body weight and memory decline has not yet been established, a number of studies suggest that watching your weight may be a good way to protect your brain.

In research using data gathered from brain scans conducted for a long-term study of cardiovascular health, scientists employed sophisticated computer techniques to analyze and compare the volume of brain structures in 94 people in their 70s. All of the participants were cognitively normal at the time the scans were done and five years later when the analysis occurred, according to a report published online August 6, 2009 in the journal *Human Brain Mapping*. The subjects were divided into three groups—those with a normal weight indicated by a body mass index (BMI) of 18.5 to 24.9, overweight individuals with a BMI of 25 to 29.9, and obese individuals with a BMI of 30 and over. (The BMI is a calculation of body fat using a person's weight in relation to height.)

The analysis showed that obese participants had brains that were eight percent smaller than participants of normal weight, and overweight participants had brains approximately six percent smaller than normal. According to the study's lead author, the brains of obese participants looked 16 years older and the brains of overweight participants looked eight years older than the brains of their normal-weight counterparts, an indication of "severe brain degeneration." The regions affected by obesity are the same brain areas involved in Alzheimer's disease (AD), the authors pointed out.

In an even larger investigation conducted several years ago, researchers who recruited 10,276 middle-age members of a California health plan and followed them for 27 years found that compared to participants with normal body weight, those who were obese had a 74 percent increased risk of dementia, and those who were overweight (but not obese) had a 35 percent increased risk. In a separate five-year study, a higher body mass index (BMI, a measurement of weight adjusted for height that is used to estimate obesity) correlated to lower scores on tests of thought-processing, attention and memory among 2,223 French men and women. An even larger investigation that looked at the relationship between weight and various forms of dementia among participants in 10 international studies suggests that people who are obese face a 42 percent increased risk of dementia compared to people with normal weight. However, the study also found that being underweight increased risk of dementia by 36 percent compared to having a normal weight.

Experts are unsure precisely what causes the association between weight and memory loss. A recent study suggests that genetic factors associated with both obesity and dementia may play a role in the relationship (see Box 8-4). Other research suggests that the effects of poor glucose tolerance—a common complication of

---

NEW FINDING

Box 8-4: Gene increases risk for both obesity and dementia

More than 33 percent of Americans carry a variant of a common gene that both increases their likelihood of obesity and makes them more vulnerable to Alzheimer's disease (AD), according to a new study published online April 19, 2010 in the *Proceedings of the National Academy of Sciences*. Researchers analyzed genetic data and brain scans of 206 healthy adults ages 55 to 90 and found that a certain form of the fat mass and obesity gene, or FTO, is associated with brain volume deficits. Images of the brains of participants with the FTO variant were eight percent more likely than images of participants without the variant to show reduction in brain volume in the frontal lobes—a region associated with decision-making—and 12 percent more likely to show atrophy of the occipital lobes of the brain—a region responsible for processing vision and other sensory perceptions. People with reduced brain volume are believed to be more susceptible to the effects of AD because they have less brain reserve available to compensate for damage associated with the disease. The effects of the gene variant can be minimized through regular exercise and a low-fat diet, the study's lead author said.

Box 8-5:
Physical strength linked to lower Alzheimer's risk

Older adults who have strong muscles may be less likely to develop Alzheimer's disease (AD) than comparable individuals who are physically weak. Researchers assessed the strength of nine muscle groups in each of 970 dementia-free men and women ages 54 to 100, and followed study participants for four years. During follow-up, 138 participants developed AD. Individuals who ranked in the top 10 percent for physical strength had a 61 percent lower risk of developing AD and a 48 percent lower risk of mild cognitive problems than those who ranked in the lowest 10 percent, the researchers reported in the November 2009 *Archives of Neurology*. The study authors believe that an underlying mechanism may cause both loss of strength and waning mental ability, and urged older people to stay physically active to help ensure good brain health.

obesity—may cause atrophy of the brain's learning and memory centers in obese individuals, and/or that low brain levels of the hormone leptin associated with obesity may be responsible for learning and memory problems. Being underweight may reflect the effects of early-stage dementia, rather than factors that may cause cognitive decline. Since research indicates that keeping your weight at healthy levels may be one way to preserve memory, consider talking with your doctor about adjusting your diet and exercise routine so you can maintain a healthy weight.

Still other research has added a further complication in efforts to understand the relationship between weight and dementia risk. While evidence suggests that obesity in mid-life is a significant risk factor for subsequent development of dementia, a recent analysis of the cognitive status of participants in the long-term Cardiovascular Health Study suggests that obesity among people over 65 may actually have a protective effect, according to a report in the March 2009 issue of *Archives of Neurology*. The study authors say their findings were "consistent with physical changes in the trajectory toward disability and frailty" and "reinforce the necessity of monitoring weight loss closely in older adults."

Exercise

Leading a sedentary lifestyle makes you more prone to cognitive decline, as well as to conditions linked to Alzheimer's, such as diabetes, high blood pressure and obesity. A good aerobic workout increases the flow of oxygen-rich blood to areas of the brain responsible for learning and memory. Exercise increases levels of brain-derived neurotrophic factor (BDNF), a chemical that protects neurons and strengthens synapses in the brain. Research suggests exercise also may spur the growth of new nerve cells in an important memory center of the brain called the hippocampus, slow age-associated declines in brain density, increase immune function in the brain, and counteract the effects of stress. Keeping muscles fit may also reduce risk of dementia, according to a recent study (see Box 8-5). Researchers found that stronger seniors were less likely to show signs of cognitive decline.

Studies show that people who are physically active have better brain functioning and a lower risk of cognitive decline and dementia (see Box 8-6). One investigation suggests that it is the improved blood flow associated with regular exercise that leads to better brain health among older adults who stay physically fit. In 2008, researchers assessed the physical fitness levels, brain blood flow, and cognitive performance of 42 women between the ages of 50 and 90, some of whom exercised regularly and some of whom did not exercise. They found that the women who were the most physically fit tended to have better blood flow to their brains during exercise and generally scored 10 percent higher on tests of memory, reasoning and thinking than women who were sedentary. The findings suggest that better blood flow to the brain translates into improved cognition, and that staying physically fit and boosting cerebral circulation may be one way for people to retain mental acuity as they age.

That suggestion is supported by a larger study comparing sedentary and active older adults that suggested that inactivity can significantly increase risk for vascular dementia (VaD), the second-most-common cause of dementia. Researchers surveyed a group of 749 men and women who were age 65 or older about their exercise habits, then followed them for four years. They found that compared to subjects who walked the least at the beginning of the study, subjects who walked the most were 73 percent less likely to develop dementia. Subjects who engaged in the most exercise of any type—including gardening, housework or bicycling—had a 76 percent lower risk of vascular dementia. The study authors suggest that exercise may improve brain health by improving blood flow, promoting the growth of new connections among brain cells, stimulating the release of beneficial brain chemicals, and providing mental and social stimulation.

If you've been inactive for a while, see your doctor about designing an exercise program that's safe for you. Aim for at least half an hour of walking, swimming or other aerobic exercise at least five days a week. Make it a point to pursue varied activities: Even household chores and gardening count as exercise. Be sure to include exercise that improves balance and coordination, and spend some time in each exercise session engaging in strength training, which boosts energy, increases muscle mass, and helps you burn fat faster.

Break bad habits

Smoking, excessive alcohol consumption and illicit drug use all have been linked to mental decline. If you smoke, talk to your doctor about smoking-cessation aids and other ways to help to you quit. The deleterious effects of smoking on the lungs and cardiovascular system are well known. Less well known, perhaps, are its consequences for the brain. The tobacco habit is thought to cause negative effects such as degeneration of the brain's fasciculus retroflexus (a bundle of nerve fibers that affects emotional control and REM sleep, among other functions), damage to neurons and cell membranes in the midbrain and cerebellar vermis (an area associated with motor functions, balance and coordination), and the death of brain cells and prevention of new cell formation in the hippocampus.

Chronic heavy drinking has been linked to brain atrophy, impaired memory and learning, diminished ability to acquire, store and retrieve information, and impaired communication among brain cells. If you drink, it's advisable to do so in moderation: Limit your drinking to one or two glasses of alcohol a day at the most (confirm

NEW FINDING

Box 8-6: Exercise lowers risk of mild cognitive impairment

A report in the January 2010 issue of the *Archives of Neurology* described a study of 1,324 older adults with a median age of 83 that compared participants with MCI to participants who had normal cognition. The researchers found that participants who had performed moderate exercise such as brisk walking, aerobics, yoga or swimming while in middle age had a 39 percent reduction in the likelihood of developing MCI, and those who had exercised in late life had a 32 percent reduction in the likelihood of developing MCI.

BOX 8-7

Medications that can impair mental functioning

Many drugs have side effects that impact the brain, including these common medications:

- Analgesics such as narcotics (including propoxyphene [Darvon]) and nonsteroidal anti-inflammatory agents

- Anticholinergic agents that treat urinary symptoms

- Antihistamines

- Antihypertensive agents including methyldopa and others

- Anti-psychotics such as Haldol, Mellaril, and Thorazine

- Anti-asthma drugs

- Benzodiazepines and other anti-anxiety and sleeping pills

- Beta blockers such as propranolol

- cardiac medications including various digitalis preparations

- Cimetidine (Tagamet)

- Glaucoma eye drops

- Hormones such as Synthroid and Thyroxin

- Lithium

- Steroids such as Prednisone

- Tricyclic antidepressants such as Elavil and Tofranil

this amount with your doctor). Avoid illicit drug use, which also can have serious negative consequences for the brain.

Manage your medications

A number of medications commonly prescribed to older adults have unwanted cognitive side effects (see Box 8-7). The more of these drugs you take, the higher the odds are that you'll see some mental decline. Because your sensitivity to the effects of drugs increases with age and medications tend to linger longer in your system, side effects can show up at lower doses than they did when you were younger.

Any decrease in cognitive function occurring soon after initiating a new drug, or soon after changing the dose of a medication you are already taking, suggests that the new drug, or new dose, is the cause of the cognitive difficulty. Check all medications you're taking, including herbal supplements and over-the-counter drugs, with your doctor. Report any unusual side effects you experience to your physician immediately.

Not all medications are bad for memory, however. Research suggests that certain medications—such as cholesterol-lowering drugs called statins and blood pressure drugs called angiotensin receptor blockers (ARBs)—may be associated with reduced risk for Alzheimer's disease or dementia.

Cholesterol-lowering statin medications such as Lipitor, Zocor, Lescol and Mevacor may halve the risk of developing dementia, Alzheimer's disease or cognitive impairment without dementia, according to a study published in the July 29, 2008 issue of *Neurology*. Researchers followed 1,674 cognitively normal men and women ages 60 and older for about five years, during which time 130 subjects developed dementia or cognitive impairment. After adjusting for factors such as smoking, genetic background and education, the scientists found that the 27 percent of study participants who had taken statin medications at some point during the study period were half as likely to develop dementia as those who did not take statins. Although the reason for the effect is not clear, one theory is that statins may help lower high insulin levels in the brain that are associated with Alzheimer's pathology. However, researchers do not suggest people take statins solely to prevent cognitive problems until more is known about the mechanisms underlying their effects on the brain.

Other common medications—a class of blood pressure medication called angiotensin receptor blockers (ARBs)—may lower risk for Alzheimer's disease (AD) and slow its progression, according to a review of the records of more than five million patients with a median age of 75 in a Veteran's Administration database. ARBs block receptors for Angiotensin II, a chemical that causes muscles surrounding blood vessels to contract, narrowing the vessels and raising blood pressure. Common ARBs include irbesartan (AVAPRO), candesartan (ATACAND), losartan (COZAAR), and valsartan (DIOVAN).The preliminary study compared patients using ARBs with those using another blood pressure medication, lisinopril, and with those using various other cardiovascular drugs. Researchers found that individuals who took ARBs were 26 percent less likely to develop AD than those who took lisinopril, and 38 percent less likely than those using other cardiovascular drugs to develop AD or other forms of dementia. Individuals with AD or dementia who took ARBs were up to 45 percent less likely to develop markers of worsening disease, such as admission to a nursing home, sundowning (a form of agitated behavior), or death. Use of ARBs also appeared to reduce neurological damage from stroke. It is thought that ARBs may help protect nerve cells from injury or promote their recovery following damage to blood vessels, the researchers said in a presentation at the 2008 International Conference on Alzheimer's Disease in Chicago.

Reduce stress

Everyone encounters stressful situations from time to time with no lasting consequences, but chronic or severe stress can take its toll on your brain. Feelings of pressure, tension, and distress increase levels of the stress hormone cortisol (see Box 8-8). Excessive or prolonged elevations in cortisol can lead to deterioration of networks of dendrites that connect neurons with one another, reducing communication among brain cells. The functioning of neurotransmitters—chemicals responsible for transmitting messages from one cell to another—is also impaired by long-term stress. The creation of new neurons in the hippocampus to replace injured or dying cells (a process called neurogenesis) may slow, resulting in the gradual shrinkage of that key memory area. Research has linked shrinkage of the hippocampus with a higher risk of Alzheimer's disease. Stress also may activate protein kinase C, a brain enzyme that can impair functioning in the prefrontal cortex, the decision-making center of the brain that is responsible for short-term memory.

Researchers at Chicago's Rush University Medical Center have found evidence that chronic psychological distress may be a risk factor for mild cognitive impairment (MCI). Using data collected on 1,256 older adults with no history of dementia, the researchers assessed subjects' proneness to distress, then tracked changes in cognitive ability over a 12-year period. They found that subjects who most often experienced negative emotions and distress were 40 percent more likely to develop mild memory problems than those who were least likely to experience these emotions.

Fortunately, there are ways to protect your brain from the harmful effects of stress and reduce your risk for memory problems. One excellent way to protect your memory is to learn techniques that help you cope during stressful times. The

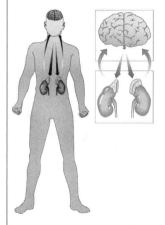

BOX 8-9

The relaxation response

1. The basic BHI relaxation response technique involves these simple steps:

2. Sit or lie comfortably in a place where you will not be disturbed.

3. Select a personal focus: A word, sound, prayer or short phrase—for example, "peace," "one," or "the Lord is my shepherd."

4. Close your eyes and progressively relax your muscles, starting at your feet and working upward to your neck and facial muscles.

5. Take deep, slow breaths, saying your focus word, sound, phrase or prayer silently to yourself as you exhale.

6. When other thoughts come to mind, gently push them away and return to silently repeating your focus word. Mentally observe interruptions, but don't worry about them. Simply return your thoughts to your focus word or phrase.

7. Continue deep breathing, word repetition, and relaxation for 10 to 20 minutes, occasionally peeking at a watch or clock to keep track of the time.

8. When your time is up, sit quietly for a minute or so. Gradually allow other thoughts to return, then open your eyes and sit for another minute before resuming your normal activities.

9. Practice the relaxation response once or twice each day, preferably before breakfast and before dinner.

Relaxation Response (see Box 8-9), a technique developed at the Benson-Henry Institute for Mind Body Medicine of Massachusetts General Hospital (BHI), has proven effective in lowering respiratory rate, blood pressure, and oxygen consumption, and may possibly help reduce levels of oxidative stress on cells as well. Other stress-reducing techniques include deep-breathing exercises, yoga, tai chi, progressive relaxation, visualization, meditation, and relaxing activities such as listening to soothing music or taking a warm bath. If you are feeling overwhelmed by stress, consider seeking help from a mental health professional.

Get adequate sleep

Getting less than six hours of sleep at night can do more than leave you feeling tired the next day—it has a significant effect on your memory. Research suggests that during restful sleep your brain consolidates newly acquired information and strengthens memories against interference. Sleep deprivation can seriously disturb cognition (see Box 8-10).

Even a short nap may help you retain information more effectively. Researchers trained 33 volunteers in a series of memory tasks that included memorizing certain words, a complex line drawing, and a maze. After training, 16 subjects took a 45-minute nap, while 17 watched a movie. Results showed that among subjects who had learned the training tasks well, napping significantly improved performance on tests of recall compared to subjects who stayed awake. Nappers

NEW FINDING

Box 8-10: Sleep loss affects remembering and quality of decisions

Recent research suggests that sleep deprivation may also lead to poor decision-making. In an effort to investigate the effects of poor sleep on various aspects of cognitive functioning, researchers observed 23 healthy adults in a controlled laboratory environment. The participants were divided into two groups, one that slept normally and one that was deprived of sleep for 62 hours. Three times during the study, participants completed batteries of tests designed to assess executive functioning, which involves the ability to initiate an action, ignore distractions while focusing on an action, and inhibit inappropriate actions. Executive function also includes basic measures like processing speed, response speed and efficiency of working memory (the type of memory involved in remembering an unfamiliar telephone number long enough to dial it). These measures have been widely assumed to be affected by sleep deprivation. The tests also assessed non-executive components of cognition, such as the ability to collect and log information. The research, published in the January 2010 issue of the journal *Sleep*, showed that sleep deprivation had little effect on working memory and other executive functions, but had significant influence on the effectiveness of non-executive functions such as remembering and interpreting important information. Participants who were sleep-deprived could make decisions, but their decisions seemed to be based on fragmentary or faulty information. Insufficient sleep seemed to affect the quality of their decisions, not their ability to make decisions and act on them.

who did not learn well performed at the level of those who stayed awake. Napping associated with excessive daytime drowsiness may indicate a sleep disorder or other medical problem that requires medical assessment. But this research suggests that for healthy people who are motivated to learn, a short snooze may help fix information in the memory and make it easier to remember.

Insufficient sleep not only interferes with memory consolidation, but also harms short-term or working memory, which is involved in temporarily storing and managing information. Lack of sleep also can make it more difficult for you to acquire memories of skills and procedures—such as how to work a computer or ride a bike. Research suggests brain changes caused by sleepiness can be reversed through non-pharmacological strategies such as exposure to bright light and manipulating body temperature. Scientists investigated the brain function of 20 older adults (average age 61) who had suffered from chronic insomnia—but no other underlying health problems—for at least 2.5 years, and compared them with 12 carefully matched subjects without insomnia. At the beginning of the investigation all participants underwent functional magnetic resonance imaging (fMRI) of their brains as they performed tests of verbal fluency. The insomnia subjects were then divided into two groups, one of whom received a six-week program of sleep therapy involving body temperature manipulations, exposure to bright light, counseling in sleep hygiene, and other interventions. The second group received no treatment. At the end of the six-week period, researchers repeated the fMRI scans while participants in both insomnia groups again performed verbal tests.

Results of the study revealed that initially, insomnia subjects showed diminished activity in the prefrontal cortical areas of their brains while performing verbal tasks compared to the control group. After six weeks, the insomnia subjects who received sleep therapy reported significantly improved sleep, and brain scans indicated they had recovered normal brain activity. The insomnia subjects who did not receive therapy experienced no improvement in brain activity. The authors of the study, which was published in the September 2008 issue of the journal *Sleep*, report non-pharmacological sleep therapy might work well for adults with chronic insomnia in clinical practice.

The quality of sleep and sleep architecture appear to change with age. Adults over 65 experience less Stage IV sleep—the deep, restorative stage of sleep—than younger people, may take longer to fall asleep, and may be easier to awaken, research shows. But regular sleep disturbance is not a normal part of aging. Individuals who experience chronic sleep problems (see Box 8-11) should seek treatment for their sleep disturbance. Seeing a doctor about conditions such as sleep apnea, restless legs syndrome, and insomnia may be a good way to address memory loss.

BOX 8-11

Do you have a sleep problem?

If you have any of the following symptoms, consider seeing your doctor about your sleep difficulties:

- Trouble falling asleep, even when you are feeling tired.

- Waking up often during the night, or having difficulty getting back to sleep once awakened.

- Awakening too early in the morning.

- Feeling fatigued and insufficiently rested when you get up in the morning.

- Experiencing daytime grogginess, drowsiness, irritability, fatigue, trouble concentrating, or difficulty performing normal activities.

- Feeling the need for sleeping pills or alcohol to get to sleep.

To get a better night's sleep and bolster your memory, establish a sensible sleep routine and stick to it. Relax quietly before going to bed, and try to retire at the same time each night and awaken at the same time each morning. Sleep in a darkened room with minimal noise. Find ways to reduce stress. Seek treatment for anxiety, medical disorders, and mood disorders that may interfere with your sleep. Limit alcohol and avoid caffeine at least four to six hours before you go to bed, and limit heavy meals and liquids in the evening. Speak with your doctor about medications you are taking that may be interfering with your sleep. Be sure to get plenty of exercise to help reduce tension and promote relaxation, but don't exercise close to bedtime. Getting outside in the sunlight for at least 10 minutes each day also may help you sleep more soundly.

Stay socially active

Research suggests that having close relationships and staying socially active is a good way to keep your memory strong and slow cognitive decline. Social interaction requires paying attention to your surroundings, following a conversation, responding to the actions of others, and watching for verbal and non-verbal cues—all of which make demands on the brain (see Box 8-12).

Several years ago, researchers at the University of Michigan assessed survey data to look at the connection between social interaction and mental functioning among 3,610 adults. They found that subjects who reported higher levels of social interaction (such as getting together with neighbors, relatives and friends, or talking on the telephone with them) performed better on tests of working memory, knowledge of personal information, and current events. The more socializing, the better the cognitive functioning, the researchers found.

Other studies have shown that people who have a positive outlook and get together with friends to enjoy social activities may be protected against dementia. After surveying 506 older adults about their lifestyle and personality traits, researchers followed the individuals for six years, during which time 144 developed some form of dementia. When investigators assessed personality traits and lifestyle along with risk of dementia, they found that people who were active, outgoing, and relaxed were more likely to be socially active and optimistic than less extroverted people, and less likely to develop dementia. "Strategies to change lifestyle, such as having an active lifestyle, engagement in different leisure activities, i.e. mental, social and physical activities, or having a rich social network, may protect against dementia," the lead author concluded.. Lack of social contact, on the other hand, seems to put people at increased risk for dementia. A well-known investigation by researchers at the University of

Chicago conducted several years ago found that people who described themselves as feeling lonely and socially isolated were twice as likely to develop dementia as people who reported being socially active. The researchers used a questionnaire to assess feelings of loneliness among 823 healthy 80-year-olds, then tested them for signs of mental confusion and memory loss over a period of four years. During the study, 76 people developed dementia. Subjects who reported feeling lonely were up to twice as likely to develop dementia as those without feelings of loneliness, and risk for dementia climbed approximately 51 percent for each additional point lonely subjects scored on the loneliness scale. Although the precise relationship between social isolation and dementia is not yet clear, it may be that loneliness triggers conditions such as elevated levels of stress hormones or high blood pressure that can cause brain changes associated with dementia.

An active social life may help protect you from dementia in other, less direct, ways. Socializing delivers many benefits, including the pleasures and enjoyment of social activities, mental stimulation that can help you stay resilient and alert, reduced stress because of reassurance and support from others, and a reduced likelihood of depression.

To keep your memory sharp, make it a point to get out with friends as often as you can, even if it's just for a quick dinner. Telephone calls, letters and e-mails to friends and loved ones also can keep you socially connected and involved with what's happening around you. If you're socially isolated, begin a campaign to win new friends by: putting yourself in new situations, such as joining a club or taking a part-time job; looking for new ways to involve yourself with others, inviting your neighbor to lunch; re-establishing contact with people you've lost touch with; and pitching in on volunteer projects (see Box 8-13). As you go about establishing a more rewarding social life, be sure to give new relationships time to develop. Resist the temptation to be overly critical or quick to judge new acquaintances; and be willing to take risks through actions such as introducing yourself, initiating conversations, or just smiling more often.

Stay mentally active

Although not as much is known about the effects of mental activity on memory as about the effects of physical activity, preliminary findings indicate that exercising your brain may be a good way to keep it sharp. Findings from animal research and several studies with human subjects indicate that occupying the brain with demanding tasks can help preserve memory and alertness, while lack of stimulation may be associated with a greater risk of developing dementia.

BOX 8-13

How to become more socially active

Try these suggestions for staying socially active:

- **Take the initiative.** Introduce yourself, speak out in group situations, and invite others to join you in social activities.

- **Reconnect.** Contact friends and family members you may have lost touch with to reestablish old ties.

- **Join a group.** Become involved with others through activities such as volunteer work, attendance at religious services, or sports activities such as water aerobics classes.

- **Meet your neighbors.** Conversations with shopkeepers, residents, and others in your neighborhood could lead to new friendships and pursuits.

- **Take up a new hobby.** In addition to being stimulating in their own right, hobbies often lead to new friendships with fellow enthusiasts.

- **Assess your living situation.** Consider relocating to be closer to family or friends with whom you enjoy spending time, or move into a community geared to older adults that provides opportunities to interact with others.

Box 8-14: Scientists find visual evidence of effects of learning on brain

A recent study uncovered the first visual evidence that mental stimulation and learning promote brain health, a finding that suggests that continued learning might help counteract some of the cognitive effects of aging in humans. Working with brain tissue and laboratory animals, the researchers found that learning stimulates the release of a protein called brain derived neurotrophic factor (BDNF) in the brain. This protein activates receptors that keep brain cells functioning optimally, and promotes the development of communication points between neurons called synapses. The BDNF effects are linked to brain waves associated with the encoding of new memories that normally become less robust as people age, the researchers said in a report published in the March 1, 2010 online edition of the *Proceedings of the National Academy of Sciences*. A principal author of the study says the discoveries "suggest that staying mentally active as we age can keep neuronal BDNF signaling at a constant rate, which may limit memory and cognitive decline.

Some research suggests that mental activity may actually reshape the brain (see Box 8-14). In one study, scientists used an electron microscope to assess the number of synapses (points of connection with other brain cells) in post-mortem brain tissue from the prefrontal cortex of 16 subjects. They found that subjects whose professions had required the greatest skill or education had 17 percent more synapses for each brain cell than subjects who had the least skill or education.

Keeping the brain stimulated with ordinary activities such as reading the paper, playing checkers or going to a play may help prevent dementia, according to a large study conducted several years ago using data from the Rush Memory and Aging Project in Chicago, a longitudinal study of more than 1,200 older people. Researchers followed a group of 775 non-demented elderly subjects for up to five years and found that those who stayed cognitively active were significantly less likely to develop dementia than those who were cognitively inactive.

The investigators administered a questionnaire to participants—who had a mean age of 80—at the beginning of the study, asking them about their social activities and how often they performed mentally stimulating activities when they were younger, and currently. They then followed up annually with a battery of cognitive tests and questions about current mental activities.

Study results suggest that keeping the brain busy helps protect it from dementia: Participants who were cognitively active were 2.6 times less likely to develop dementia than participants who engaged in cognitive activities infrequently. They also were less likely to develop mild cognitive impairment and experienced less rapid decline in cognitive function. Post-mortem studies of the brains of 102 participants who died over the course of the investigation found no association between the level of mental activity and pathological lesions in the brain that are typical of dementia, suggesting that lack of mental activity was not a consequence of Alzheimer's disease or other dementia.

Another study presented in May 2009 at the 61st annual meeting of the American Academy of Neurology in Seattle found that mental activity may cut the risk of developing dementia in half. A study assessing the daily activities of nearly 1,300 older adults ages 70 to 89 suggests that staying mentally active may help people ward off memory loss. Researchers asked study participants, 200 of whom had been diagnosed with memory loss, to describe their activities within the past year, and in the years when they were between the ages of 50 and 65. They found that people who reported engaging in simple mental activities such as playing games, using the computer, reading books and doing crafts or hobbies in their later years experienced a 30 to 50 percent decreased risk of developing memory loss compared to individuals who did not engage in those activities. Similarly, people who watched television for less than seven hours a day were half as likely to develop memory problems as people who spent their later years watching TV seven hours or more each day. Mid-life activities such as reading magazines and socializing lowered the risk for memory loss later in life by 40 percent.

Even when stimulating activities are pursued at an older age after a lifetime of little mental stimulation they may help boost brain reserve and decrease risk of dementia, some research shows. Activities that require concentration, involve as many of the senses as possible, and involve new or unexpected experiences and approaches are especially stimulating to the brain.

There are many ways to integrate mental stimulation into your day. Challenge your mind with crossword puzzles, brain teasers, math problems or sudoku puzzles. Learn a favorite quotation by heart, stock up on funny jokes to tell your friends, or commit your shopping list to memory. Play card games—alone or with friends—or challenge family members to a game of Scrabble, chess, bridge or poker. Read newspapers and magazines to keep up with current events, and write letters or keep a journal. Try new hobbies, take a class at the local college, or learn a new language. Even changing your routine from time to time can be mentally stimulating.

Protect your brain

Several studies have suggested that a head injury may increase your risk for dementia. Traumatic brain injury (TBI) caused by a blow to the head, a fall, or even violent jarring may injure sensitive brain tissues in ways that might cause later declines in cognition. Between 400,000 and 500,000 Americans are hospitalized every year for head injury. Most of these injuries are caused by motor vehicle accidents (50 percent) and falls (21 percent). Symptoms vary depending on the area of the brain affected by the injury, and may not show up until hours, days or even weeks later (see Box 8-15). Prompt medical treatment may help prevent further damage to vulnerable tissues.

Although further research is necessary to clarify the precise relationship between TBI and later dementia, taking steps to protect yourself from possible head injury is a wise precaution. Some common-sense suggestions: use your seatbelt when you drive or ride in a car; check your home for fall hazards (such as loose rugs or loose electrical cords) and eliminate them; wear appropriate footwear, such as non-slip boots for icy weather; have your doctor recommend exercises that can improve your muscle strength, gait, and sense of balance; wear a helmet to protect your head while riding a bike or engaging in other activities that carry a risk of head injury; and check with your doctor to see if you can change medications that cause you to become drowsy or dizzy. ■

BOX 8-15

Symptoms of traumatic brain injury

The Centers for Disease Control and Prevention recommends calling the doctor immediately if you notice any of these symptoms following a blow or jolt to the head:

- Headaches or neck pain that won't go away
- Trouble with mental tasks such as remembering, concentrating, or decision-making
- Slow thinking, speaking, acting or reading
- Changes in sleep patterns (sleeping a lot more or having a hard time sleeping)
- Getting lost or easily confused
- Mood changes (feeling sad or angry for no reason)
- Feeling tired all the time, lacking energy or motivation
- Feeling light-headed or dizzy, or losing balance
- An urge to vomit (nausea)
- Increased sensitivity to lights, sounds or distractions
- Blurred vision or eyes that tire easily
- Loss of sense of smell or taste
- Ringing in the ears

9 STRATEGIES TO HELP BOOST MEMORY

Some degree of memory loss is an inevitable part of the aging process. The good news is that there are simple strategies that can help you improve your ability to remember things. Try some of the suggestions in this chapter to increase your ability to focus on information, fix it in your mind, and recall it more easily when you wish to.

Learn basic memory skills

These simple approaches will help make information easier to retain and recall:

- Acknowledge memory problems. Accepting the need to compensate for memory challenges and taking steps to adapt to a faltering memory can help reduce frustration and stress.

- Get motivated. To remember something, you have to make an effort. Think how the information will be useful to you, so that you are motivated to remember. For example, memorizing your doctor's telephone number is useful because it can spare you from having to search for the number in an emergency.

- Concentrate. Focus on each memory task one at a time. Divided attention impairs your ability to fix information in your mind.

- Get organized. The more organized you are, the better you'll be able to concentrate on what you need to remember. Always keep important, frequently used belongings such as your house keys and your wallet in the same place. Make regular use of a calendar, bulletin board, electronic organizer or some other device to keep track of your appointments and other important dates. Use medication dispensers to help you remember to take your pills.

- Use mnemonic strategies and other memory techniques. Organize information into rhymes, acronyms or other forms that are easier for your brain to encode or recall. For example, to remember the date of Christopher Columbus's famous voyage, people often use the mnemonic phrase, "In 1492, Columbus sailed the ocean blue." Practice puzzles or memorization games to strengthen your memory.

- Manage your memory. Break the information you want to remember into small pieces so that you don't overload your memory. Also take breaks during the process of remembering to give your brain a rest.

- Associate. Connect new bits of information with things you've already learned. For example, if you meet someone new who is named Sandra, ask yourself whether you know anyone else with the same name. The association may help you remember the name of your new acquaintance the next time you meet.

■ Make sure you understand the information you are trying to remember. You'll be more likely to remember the steps you must take to successfully plant a sapling if you understand the reasons for them.

■ Use cues. Put your empty medicine bottle by the door to remind yourself to fill your prescription. Paste a "sticky note" on the refrigerator to help you remember to buy milk. Use clocks with timers to help you remember to turn off the oven.

■ Train, rehearse, practice. For example, if you find you have trouble concentrating, practice focusing on one subject or task for 10 minutes without letting your mind stray. The next day, increase your concentration time to 12 or 15 minutes, gradually building your ability to focus and ignore distractions. Or read a book with the television on to challenge your powers of concentration. Try playing brain-training games on the internet to boost your brain's processing speed. Memorize your favorite poems, or learn to play a new piece on the piano.

■ Lean on others. Ask your friends or family to help you remember important appointments or tasks.

For a handy way to remember key memory strategies, see Box 9-1.

Use mindfulness meditation

Research suggests that the ability to pay attention—a key aspect of remembering—declines with age. One excellent way to improve your ability to pay attention and remember is to practice mindfulness meditation. This form of meditation involves focusing awareness on sensory stimuli in the present moment, while ignoring intrusive thoughts and inner chatter.

The work of Massachusetts General Hospital neuroscientist Sara Lazar, PhD, has demonstrated that cortical regions of the brain important to memory are preserved in older individuals who meditate. These regions, which are responsible for attention, sensory processing and integrating emotional and cognitive processes, normally thin with aging. In people who practice mindfulness meditation, the regions remain thick, an indication that performance of cognitive tasks associated with those regions has not declined.

Mindfulness meditation can help slow a racing mind, allow for paying attention to information and learning, and improve the ability to focus on information without becoming distracted and jumping from thought to thought. Recent research

Box 9-2: Regular meditation may reverse memory loss

Results of a small study of 15 older adults with memory problems suggest that daily 12-minute meditation sessions over a period of eight weeks can improve overall memory function. (See a description of a simple meditation technique in Box 9-3.) The participants experienced increased blood flow to brain regions involved in memory retrieval and improved their scores on tests of general memory, attention, and cognition. Their performance on a test requiring them to name as many animals as they could in one minute also improved. A control group of comparable adults who listened to violin concertos for 12 minutes a day showed no significant increases in blood flow or improvements in cognition, according to a report in the April 2010 *Journal of Alzheimer's Disease*.

suggests it may even help reverse memory loss (see Box 9-2). However, it is necessary to practice mindfulness meditation regularly to experience its benefits. A routine of daily meditation lasting for a 20 minutes is sufficient (see Box 9-3).

Make a weekly plan

A weekly plan in which you note your goals, activities, appointments, and chores for each day of the week can help you stay on track without cluttering your mind with minutia. Try to draw up your plan at a regular time each week, using a weekly calendar or appointment book with enough space for writing information. Divide items into categories, such as "home," "social activities," "medical," and "shopping." First, check last week's schedule and carry over any tasks you have not completed. Then look over important papers to note letters that must be answered, bills that need to be paid, telephone calls that must be made, and so on. Think of tasks you need to accomplish, and projects you want to concentrate on for the week. Make a simple plan including entries such as:

- Appointments
- Chores
- Purchases you need to make
- Social events
- Special dates such as birthdays or anniversaries
- Exercise activities
- Routine maintenance on your car or home
- Medical reminders

As new tasks arise, get in the habit of recording them in your weekly plan so that important information will be readily accessible. Cross off items you've accomplished to help you keep track of what still needs to be done.

At the beginning of each day, consult your weekly plan. If you wish, use a pocket-sized notebook to note that day's appointments and chores and carry the notebook with you so you needn't worry about forgetting an important obligation or task.

Make information stand out

A study published in the November 2008 issue of *Psychological Science* suggests that it is confusion with previously learned information rather than the passage of time that weakens memory traces and interferes with their transfer to long-term storage. That means you may be able to increase you ability to retain a memory by endowing the information with unique elements or associations so that it stands apart from other information you may be exposed to around the same time. You can use a number of imaginative techniques to make things you want to remember distinctive. Some suggestions:

- **Take a snapshot:** Take a moment to make a complete visual record of what you want to remember, noticing as many details as possible. Deliberately focus your attention, creating a mental "photograph" that will stand out in your mind.

- **Prepare a speech:** Pretend you must describe or explain the information you want to remember to someone else. Rehearsing details—especially if you do so out loud—will help fix them in your mind.

- **Sing it:** Make up a musical ditty that contains the information you're trying to remember such as a shopping list. The rhythm and tune of your jingle will help fix the information in your mind so you can recall it more easily later on.

- **Create a vivid mental image:** For example, to help you remember to buy peanut butter, spaghetti and olives at the supermarket, try picturing yourself with peanut butter smeared in your hair, a necklace of olives and a hula skirt made of spaghetti strands. The vivid image should make your shopping list easy to recall. ■

10 GETTING HELP FOR MEMORY PROBLEMS

When memory problems start to interfere with your daily life, it may be time to call a specialist. This list can help you sort out the different types of professionals who treat memory problems:

■ **Geriatric psychiatrists (MDs):** These physicians specialize in older adults. Their extensive medical training has given them a thorough knowledge of the body's functions and the complex relationship between emotional illness and other medical illnesses in older individuals. They are well qualified to distinguish between physical and psychological causes of both mental and physical disorders and are expert at dealing with memory problems that involve psychiatric issues such as major depression, anxiety, agitation, or psychotic symptoms such as delusions.

■ **Geriatric psychologists (PhDs):** Geriatric psychologists hold PhD degrees in psychology. Since their specialty involves the psychological assessment and treatment of mental and nervous disorders associated with the senior years as distinct from physical ailments, they largely focus on issues involving memory, competency, depression, anxiety, or adjustment difficulties. Through testing and therapy, they help older adults who experience anxiety, depression, or other psychological problems associated with memory loss.

■ **Geriatricians (MDs):** These physicians specialize in promoting the health of older adults and in preventing and treating disease and disability associated with later life. They treat Alzheimer's disease, as well as the complex medical issues that may complicate memory problems in older adults, such as Parkinson's disease, cardiovascular issues or chronic pulmonary disease.

■ **Neurologists (MDs):** These specially trained physicians diagnose and treat disorders of the nervous system. They focus on diseases of the brain, spinal cord, nerves, and nerve centers, and are often consulted by individuals needing assessment of neurological and memory problems such as Parkinson's disease, multiple sclerosis and Alzheimer's disease. Because neurologists are experts in neurological structures, they are especially knowledgeable about the various regions of the brain and their role in physical and mental functioning.

Research trials

Another excellent option for treatment of memory disorders is enrolling in a research trial offered by major medical institutions in your area. A clinical trial is a research study that uses human volunteers in a highly safe and controlled manner to answer specific medical questions about new therapies. Clinical trials make it possible for individuals with memory disorders to benefit from new treatments while contributing to medical knowledge.

People who enroll in clinical trials may benefit from their participation, but they also must be aware that there is risk, since these treatments are not yet validated. Trials offer options not yet available in most treatment settings and give people the opportunity to receive cutting-edge therapies with excellent care. Personal contact with medical researchers also helps inform people about the latest medical advances. And participating in a clinical trial gives you an opportunity to help improve the health of others who might benefit from new treatments in the future.

If you are considering this option, you can find out about clinical trials in your area by contacting the following excellent sources of information on current studies:

- **The federal government** maintains a computer database of clinical trials that provides information on many studies at no cost. The database can be accessed online at http://clinicaltrials.gov.

- **Patient Recruitment and Public Liaison Office Clinical Center**

  National Institutes of Health, Building 61, 10 Cloister Court

  Bethesda, MD 20892-4754

  (800) 411-1222

  www.cc.nih.gov/ccc/prpl

- **Alzheimer's Disease Clinical Trials Database**

  Sponsored by the U.S. Food and Drug Administration (FDA) and the National Institute on Aging

  www.alzheimers.org/trials

A Boston-based publishing and information services company called CenterWatch provides an extensive list of clinical trials being conducted internationally that have been approved by the Independent Review Board (IRB), a committee empowered by the FDA to assess and approve research on human subjects.

- **CenterWatch**

  100 N. Washington St., Suite 301

  Boston, MA 02114

  Phone: (617) 948-5100

  Fax: (617) 948-5101

  www.centerwatch.com/patient/trials.html

Professional organizations and support groups

There are a number of excellent professional organizations and support groups that help people with dementia and Alzheimer's. These groups are a free source of information, support, referrals, and other services that can be invaluable to people with memory problems and their families. Among the better-known groups are:

Administration on Aging
Washington, DC 20201
Phone: 202-619-0724
www.aoa.dhhs.gov

Alzheimer's Association
National Office
225 N. Michigan Ave., Fl. 17
Chicago, IL 60601
24/7 Helpline: 800-272-3900
www.alz.org/overview.asp

American Heart Association
National Center
7272 Greenville Avenue
Dallas, TX 75231
Phone: 800-242-8721
www.americanheart.org

American Psychiatric Association
1000 Wilson Boulevard, Suite 1825
Arlington, Va. 22209-3901
Phone: 703-907-7300
www.psych.org

American Stroke Association
National Center
7272 Greenville Avenue
Dallas TX 75231
Phone: 888-478-7653
www.strokeassociation.org

National Institute of
Mental Health (NIMH)
Public Information and
Communications Branch
6001 Executive Boulevard,
Room 8184, MSC 9663
Bethesda, MD 20892-9663
Phone: 866-615-6464 (toll-free);
866-415-8051 (TTY toll-free)
www.nimh.nih.gov

National Institute on Aging
Building 31, Room 5C27
31 Center Drive, MSC 2292
Bethesda, MD 20892
Phone: 301-496-1752
TTY: 800-222-4225
www.nia.nih.gov

National Mental Health Association
2000 N. Beauregard Street, 6th Floor
Alexandria, Virginia 22311
Phone: 800-969-6642;
800-433-5959 (TTY)
www.nmha.org

NIH Neurological Institute
P.O. Box 5801
Bethesda, MD 20824
Phone: 800-352-9424;
301-468-5981 (TTY)
www.nids.nih.gov

National Parkinson Foundation
1501 N.W. 9th Avenue / Bob Hope Road
Miami, Florida 33136-1494
Phone: 800-327-4545
www.parkinson.org

U.S. Department of Health
& Human Services
200 Independence Avenue, SW
Washington, DC 20201
Phone: 877-696-6775
www.hhs.gov